Dedicated to the
nurses who try to see the "world" of the hospital
through the eyes of the pediatric patient.

To my children Jane, Thomas, and Timothy.
JTN

To my loving family, Charles, Colleen, Greg, and Jacqui,
and to the pediatrician who has been
my inspiration, Kathleen R. Montemayor, MD.
GRS

Table of Contents

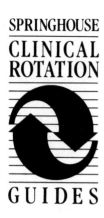

SPRINGHOUSE
**CLINICAL
ROTATION**

GUIDES

PEDIATRIC NURSING

Joan T. Newman, RN, BS, MSN
Geraldine R. Scott, RN, BS, MEd, ARNP

Springhouse Corporation
Springhouse, Pennsylvania

Staff For This Volume

Executive Director, Editorial
Stanley Loeb

Executive Director, Creative Services
Jean Robinson

Director of Trade and Textbooks
Minnie B. Rose, RN, BSN, MEd

Art Director
John Hubbard

Editorial Manager
Kevin Law

Editors
Diane Labus, Bernadette Glenn (associate acquisitions)

Copy Editor
Keith de Pinho

Designers
Stephanie Peters (associate art director), Lorraine Carbo

Art Production
Robert Perry (manager), Anna Brindisi, Donald Knauss, Christine McKinley, Robert Wieder

Typography
David Kosten (manager), Diane Paluba (assistant manager), Joyce Rossi Biletz, Brenda Mayer, Robin Rantz, Brent Rinedoller, Valerie Rosenberger

Manufacturing
Deborah Meiris (manager), T.A. Landis

Project Coordination
Aline S. Miller (manager), Laurie J. Sander

Printed in the United States of America

CRG6-010789

Library of Congress Cataloging-in-Publication Data
Newman, Joan T.
    Pediatric nursing/Joan T. Newman, Geraldine R. Scott.
      p. cm.—(Springhouse clinical rotation guides)
    Bibliography: p.
    Includes index.
    1. Pediatric nursing—Handbooks, manuals, etc.   I. Scott, Geraldine R.
    II. Title.   III. Series: Clinical rotation guides.
    [DNLM: 1. Pediatric Nursing.   WY 159 N553p]
RJ245.N49   1990
610.73′62—dc20
DNLM/DLC
for Library of Congress   89-10091
ISBN 0-87434-206-6   CIP

Special Acknowledgment

The series editor wishes to thank Florida Hospital, Orlando, Fla., owned and operated by the Adventist Health System, for the services and support that made this series possible.

Series Consulting Editor
Mary Jane Evans, RN, BSN, CCRN
Independent Consultant for Nursing Education

Advisory Board

Pediatric Nursing

Marie Scott Brown, RN, Phd, PNP
Professor of Family Nursing, School of Nursing
Oregon Health Science University
Portland, Ore.

Lillian S. Brunner, RN, MSN, ScD, LittD, FAAN
Nurse-Author
Brunner Associates, Inc.
Berwyn, Pa.

Susan B. Dickey, RNC, MSN
Assistant Professor
Department of Nursing, College of Allied Health Practice
Temple University
Philadelphia, Pa.;
Relief Staff Nurse
Children's Hospital of Philadelphia
Philadelphia, Pa.

Marilyn L. Evans, RN, PhD
Associate Professor
University of North Carolina at Greensboro
Greensboro, N.C.

Joan Holter Gildea, RNC, MA
Independent Pediatric Nursing Consultant
Darien, Connecticut;
Former Clinical Assistant Director of Nursing
New York University Medical Center
New York City, N.Y.

Celestine B. Mason, RN, BSN, MA
Nursing Care Consultant
Good Samaritan Hospital
Puyallup, Wash.;
Former Associate Professor of Nursing
Pacific Lutheran University
Tacoma, Wash.

Carol E. Smith, RN, PhD
Professor, School of Nursing
University of Kansas
Kansas City, Kan.

Kathleen Morgan Speer, RN, MSN, PhD
Associate Professor
Midwestern State University
Wichita Falls, Tex.;
Research Coordinator
Children's Medical Center
Dallas, Tex.

Preface

This book, designed as a supplementary aid, will assist the student in planning and implementing nursing care of the pediatric patient in the clinical setting. It in no way substitutes for an in-depth study of pediatric patient care; rather, its purpose is to provide quick, easy access to information useful to nursing students on pediatric clinical rotations. Within this book, the student will find clinical instruction on:

• understanding the developmental framework and related aspects of care of the pediatric patient

• performing a pediatric admission assessment and providing ongoing observation and evaluation

• identifying common pediatric-related diseases and disorders and formulating associated nursing diagnoses and interventions

• adapting procedures and diagnostic tests to the pediatric patient

• understanding the purpose and usefulness of special pediatric equipment

• caring for the pediatric surgical patient, both preoperatively and postoperatively

• recognizing signs of pediatric abuse and neglect

• giving cardiopulmonary resuscitation to infants and children.

1 Pediatric Assessment

Contrary to a common misconception, children are not miniature adults. They differ greatly from adults, both physiologically and psychologically, providing the basis for the speciality of pediatric nursing.

Your success during your assignment to the pediatric unit will depend to a great extent on your understanding of developmental variations anticipated in different age-groups. This section provides information on the developmental framework as well as essential information on obtaining a pediatric admission assessment.

☐ Developmental framework

The following developmental framework provides a concise explanation of the physical and psychosocial characteristics of children in various age-groups. (Keep in mind, however, that because each child is an individual, you can never predict exactly how a child will behave simply by noting his age.) This framework also includes nursing assessment tips related to the child's developmental age.

Neonatal period

The neonatal period extends from birth until age 1 month.

Physical characteristics

Weight. Birth weight usually varies between 5½ and 9½ lb (2,500 to 4,300 g), averaging somewhere between 7 and 7½ lb (3,200 to 3,400 g). During the first 3 to 4 days postpartum, a newborn can be expected to lose up to 10% of his body weight. (He typically regains this weight within 2 weeks.) Reassure caregivers that this is normal.

Length. The newborn's length is normally between 19″ and 21″ (48 to 53 cm).

Head. At birth, the head is normally one fourth the total body length. Head circumference ranges from 12½″ to 14″ (31.8 to 35.6 cm). At this age, skull bones are not united and sutures may be overlapping. The anterior fontanelle is diamond-shaped; the posterior fontanelle, triangular. Neither fontanelle may be palpable for several days because of molding. The newborn will lift his head when placed in a prone postition for a short time (a normal reflex).

Neck. The newborn's neck muscles are too weak to support his head. Support the head when lifting or holding him.

Chest. The chest is rounded. Breast engorgement caused by maternal hormones may occur in newborns of either sex; reassure caregivers that this is normal.

Abdomen. The abdomen is protuberant and moves with breathing.

Extremities. Hands usually are closed-fisted; arms and legs, flexed. Acrocyanosis (bluish discoloration of the hands and feet) may be present; reassure caregivers that this is normal. Movements are generalized and purposeless.

Back. The spine should be straight with no evidence of a pilonidal dimple.

Skin. Color varies with ethnicity. Most newborns have thin, delicate skin. Blood vessels usually are visible; mottling will occur when the newborn is chilled. Reddened areas over the eyelids, center of brow, and back of the neck ("stork bites") may be apparent. Mongolian spots (a bluish discoloration on the lower back and buttocks) commonly occurs in dark-skinned newborns; reassure caregivers that this is normal and will fade with time.

Daily bathing helps maintain skin integrity. Soaps recommended by the American Academy of Pediatrics include Dove, Tone, and Caress. Wrap the newborn in a blanket after bathing to provide warmth and security.

Temperature. Newborns usually have an unstable body temperature—an immature reaction to environmental extremes. To prevent appreciable heat loss from the head, keep the head covered. To further conserve body heat, dress the newborn slightly warmer than an adult. Booties provide warmth and comfort.

Sleep pattern. Because a newborn typically sleeps 18 to 20 hours a day, maintain an environment conducive to sleep.

Elimination. A newborn voids often and requires frequent diaper changes. Stools, which vary in frequency, are usually pale yellow to light brown and of a pasty consistency. When washing the diaper area, always rinse the area well and pat it dry. Commercially prepared wipes are a good alternative; however, some contain irritants.

Psychosocial characteristics
A newborn's temperament is highly individualized; support caregivers in their acceptance of this individuality. Personality and emotional development are described by Erikson's stage of trust versus mistrust (in which infants learn to trust the adults who care for them). Newborns have no wants, only needs; meeting those needs promptly and consistently builds trust.

Crying is the newborn's only means of communication. A lusty cry communicates hunger, wetness, or a lack of comfort. Investigate crying promptly.

Nursing considerations

Medication. Newborns suck reflexively; use this natural behavior to best advantage by giving medications via a nipple. This is easier to accomplish when the newborn is hungry. Another normal reflex, tongue extrusion, requires that you medicate the newborn by placing a syringe or dropper (if necessary) along the side and near the back of his mouth.

Because newborns cannot handle a large volume of fluid and may choke or drool, be sure to give small amounts of medication at a time. Also remember that a newborn's gross motor control is poor, so be sure to restrain his arms to prevent random movements and spillage.

Nutrition. When feeding the newborn, keep in mind that his normal schedule is "on demand." Formula feeding usually is scheduled every 3 to 4 hours around the clock; breast-feeding, every 2 to 3 hours.

Breast milk and commercially prepared infant formula provide total nutrition. Newborns require 50 calories per lb (110 calories per kg) of body weight every 24 hours. Breast milk and most infant formulas contain 20 calories per oz (see *Common nutritional sources for infants,* page 4, for a comparison).

Keep in mind the following:

• Never prop a bottle in the newborn's mouth; rather, hold the infant in a natural breast-feeding position.

• Encourage the mother to use a breast pump if she is unable to breast-feed the child during his regular feeding time.

• Discourage the addition of other foods to the newborn's diet.

• Remember that providing nutrition is only one aspect of feeding; feeding also provides the newborn with much-needed physical and eye contact.

• A pause in sucking indicates that the newborn needs to burp. When this occurs, bring the newborn to an upright position to allow the air bubble to rise. Be sure to pat or massage his back gently while waiting for him to burp. Then observe for regurgitation.

• A sick or small newborn may be a poor feeder. Remember that he may need to be awakened to feed on schedule. Stimulate the suck reflex by manipulating the nipple in his mouth. Also, unwrap his blanket to provide environmental stimulus; however, avoid exposing him to chills.

Safety concerns. Because a newborn tends to wiggle and squirm, be sure to keep your hands on him at all times when the crib rail is down or the Isolette is open. The gap between the crib side and the mattress must be no larger than the width of a finger. Fill any larger gaps with a blanket roll.

COMMON NUTRITIONAL SOURCES FOR INFANTS

The following list of nutritional sources is not intended as an exhaustive list. Special preparations for infants on low-sodium, low-phenyl-alaline, carbohydrate-free, and other special diets are also commercially available.

Although common formulas usually contain 20 calories/oz with standard dilution, these formulas may be diluted to other variations, according to doctor's instructions. Some formulas are available in ready-to-feed preparations of 13, 24, or 27 calories/oz.

Product name	Standard dilution	Carbohy-drate source	Protein source	Fat source	Indications for use
Enfamil	20 calories/ oz	Lactose	Casein, whey	Soy, coconut oil	Routine feed-ing
Enfamil Pre-mature	24 calories/ oz	Lactose, glu-cose poly-mers	Whey, casein	Medium-chain triglyceride, corn oil, coco-nut oil	Low birth weight
Human breast milk	Approxi-mately 20 calories/oz	Lactose	Lactalbumin, casein	Human milk fat	Routine feed-ing
Isomil, Isomil SF	20 calories/ oz	Sucrose, glu-cose poly-mers	Soy protein	Coconut oil, soy oil	Intolerance to lactose or cow's milk; diarrhea
Nursoy	20 calories/ oz	Sucrose	Soy protein	Soy oils	Sensitivity to milk protein
Nutramigen	20 calories/ oz	Sucrose, tapioca starch	Casein hydro-lysate	Corn oils	Galactosemia, intolerance to food proteins
"preemie" SMA	24 calories/ oz	Lactose, glu-cose poly-mers	Whey, casein	Medium-chain triglyceride, oleomargarine, oleic acid, co-conut oil, soy oil	Low birth weight
Pregestimil	20 calories/ oz	Corn syrup solids, tap-ioca starch	Casein hydroly-sate, L-cystine, L-tyrosine, L-tryptophan	Medium-chain triglyceride, corn oil	Malabsorption syndrome
ProSobee	20 calories/ oz	Corn syrup solids	Soy protein isolate, methi-onine	Soy oil, coco-nut oil	Sensitivity to milk protein; diarrhea
Similac with Iron	20 calories/ oz	Lactose	Casein, whey	Soy oil, coco-nut oil	Routine feed-ing
SMA Iron For-tified	20 calories/ oz	Lactose	Whey, casein	Coconut oil, safflower oil	Routine feed-ing

Other safety measures include the following:
• Position the newborn on his right side or abdomen after feeding. Watch for regurgitation and intervene to prevent aspiration.
• Because certain infant toys may hurt the newborn, be sure to check all toys for potential hazards.
• When carrying the newborn, protect him against injury by shielding his head with your hand.

Participation of the primary caregiver. Assess the caregiver's interaction with the newborn, noting eye contact, gentleness, verbal expressions, and body language. Model desirable behaviors for the caregiver by smiling, speaking softly, and holding and touching the newborn gently during your assessment.

Also assess the caregiver's needs, coping skills, support systems, and understanding of the newborn's present illness by asking questions and listening attentively. The caregiver may be frightened to touch the child, feeling too insecure or inadequate to deal with the illness. Encourage the caregiver to touch and hold the newborn and to respond promptly to his cry, stressing that conserving energy is essential for a sick infant. Offer reassurance and support by remaining at the bedside while the caregiver meets the infant's needs. To prevent the caregiver's feeling abandoned, avoid leaving the caregiver alone with the sick child. (Keep in mind that the caregiver's confidence will develop through experience.)

Infant period

Infancy extends from age 1 month to 1 year.

Physical characteristics

Growth. Infants grow rapidly, especially during the first 6 months. Weight doubles by age 5 months (with weight gain averaging about 1½ lb [680 g] per month) and triples by age 1 year.

Height normally increases 1″ (2.5 cm) per month during the first 6 months, then one half that rate during the next 6 months. By age 1 year, the infant's height will have increased by 50% over his birth height.

Head circumference normally increases ½″ (1.3 cm) per month during the first 6 months, then one half that rate during the next 6 months. By age 1 year, head circumference will have increased by one third over the circumference at birth.

The posterior fontanelle should fuse completely within 6 to 8 weeks, whereas the anterior fontanelle will remain open and diamond-shaped; measurements must be graphed and compared to normal growth percentiles (see "Physical Growth Charts" in the Appendices). Brain maturation during this period is dramatic.

Visual acuity. Visual acuity improves gradually during infancy. Convergence and binocular fixation occur by age 3 months, accommodation to near objects by age 5 months, and fixation on small objects by age 10 months (see *Visual acuity: What's normal?*).

Hearing. Hearing, which is present before birth, can be tested by checking the infant's response to a loud noise (startle reflex). By age 4 months, an infant can locate sound by turning his head to look and listen. By age 10 months, he responds to someone speaking his name; by age 1 year, he listens for recurrence of familiar sounds.

Chest. During infancy, the chest begins to take on more of an adult contour. Chest circumference will equal head circumference by age 1 year.

Motor development. A highly individualized, progressive process, motor development is marked by gradual increases in strength. During infancy, voluntary purposeful movements replace primitive reflexes. As a newborn, the child can momentarily hold his head in midline and turn his head from side to side when prone. He also may roll over accidentally. By age 4 months, he can lift his head and the anterior portion of his chest 90 degrees and can roll from his back to his side. By age 6 months, he can turn at will.

Sitting follows progressive head control. At age 6 months, the infant lifts his head when pulled to a sitting position and may be propped up to sit. Usually, by age 7 months, he can sit alone. By age 10 months, he can maneuver from a prone to a sitting position. During this period, he should be propped in a sitting position to stimulate interest in his environment.

Locomotion. By age 6 or 7 months, the infant can bear his weight when placed in a standing position. By age 9 months, he usually can pull himself to a standing position while holding onto something for balance. By age 11 months, he usually can creep on his hands and knees and can maneuver while standing and holding onto furniture. By age 1 year, he usually can walk with someone holding his hand. During this period, the infant should be allowed opportunities to experience mobility; urge caregivers to encourage development in each stage.

Fine motor development. The infant grasps reflexively from birth and observes and plays with his hands by age 4 months. By age 5 months, the grasp reflex is replaced with voluntary control. By age 8 to 10 months, the infant's crude pincer (clawing) movements develop into neat prehension (fine grasping).

During this stage, the infant should be provided with crib toys that stimulate him to reach out and grasp. When placed in a high chair for meals, he should be given food that has been cut into small pieces to encourage independent feeding.

Sleep pattern. Usually, the infant develops nocturnal sleep patterns by age 3 months. By age 6 months, he should sleep

VISUAL ACUITY: WHAT'S NORMAL?

As you probably know, a child doesn't develop 20/20 vision until he's nearly school age. How clearly should a younger child be able to see? Use the chart at right as a guide.

Age	Visual acuity
Newborn	20/300
4 to 5 months	20/200
11 to 12 months	20/100
1½ to 2 years	20/40
3 to 4 years	20/30
5 to 6 years	20/20

through the night. The infant will nap, depending on his needs. By age 8 or 9 months, he will probably need only one or two naps during the day.

The infant's sleep pattern is established by the spacing of feedings, which is related to his hunger rhythm and stomach capacity. Inform caregivers about this sleep-awake (feeding) pattern and encourage them to plan the infant's care to allow for periods of uninterrupted sleep.

Elimination. Infants usually have rapid peristaltic activity. Generally, the smaller the infant, the more often his hunger symptoms and associated defecation will occur.

Stool patterns vary, depending on the infant's diet and other related factors. Advise caregivers to check the consistency of stools before becoming overly concerned about diarrhea or constipation. Stools of breast-fed infants usually are pasty, whereas stools of formula-fed infants are firmer in consistency.

Psychosocial characteristics

Developing trust. According to Erikson's theory, the infant acquires a sense of trust through the ongoing experience of having his needs consistently met. He needs to feel physical comfort and a sense of security, the crucial element being the quality of the caregiver-child relationship. The infant needs prompt responses to his signals of distress; delayed gratification of his needs leads to mistrust.

Encourage caregivers to stay with the infant in the hospital or to visit daily to institute early bonding. Also encourage them to touch the infant when they cannot hold him.

By age 6 to 8 months, the infant shows signs of anxiety around strangers. During this time, he should be approached gently and quietly to allay apprehension. Eye contact is important.

Play. Considered by many to be the "work of the child," play (particularly through stimulation activities involving motor skills, language, and personal and social skills) is as important to developmental growth as nutrition is to physical growth.

Infants need to be played with—not just allowed to play. Knowledge of developmental milestones allows caregivers to provide appropriate forms of play; instruct caregivers, if necessary, in proper play techniques. Interventions that encourage the achievement of developmental milestones should be used. For example, an infant approaching the stage for rolling over may be stimulated by the caregiver's placing an enticing toy beside the child. However, pushing the infant beyond his capacity for learning to play will only lead to tension, frustration, and insecurity.

Keep in mind that sickness and hospitalization thwart the normal developmental growth process that occurs through play. Remember to incorporate playfulness into routine nursing care measures, such as by allowing the child to touch and manipulate equipment during the assessment procedure.

Temperament. Each infant has a unique behavioral style that affects all aspects of his developmental growth and care. For example, an infant considered to be a difficult child does better with scheduled feedings and structured caregiving routines. An infant who is considered highly distractible responds well to such soothing actions as stroking, rocking, and swinging. An infant who is considered highly active has an increased need for motor activity and needs to be watched more carefully to prevent accidents.

Understanding the variations in infant temperament helps caregivers accept and better deal with the infant's behavior. Keep in mind that caregivers may need demonstration of appropriate coping techniques.

Cognition. According to Piaget's sensorimotor phase (in which the infant differentiates himself from objects), by age 4 months, the infant begins to recognize that a stimulus initiates a chain of events. He begins using voluntary actions instead of reflexive behavior. For instance, sucking and grasping become deliberate acts. During this time, an infant who cannot feed by sucking should be given a pacifier.

By age 4 to 8 months, the infant's actions usually are repeated and more prolonged. He resorts to shaking, banging, pulling, and imitating. In play, he finds pleasure in learning new skills. He also remembers objects beyond his immediate range of vision or touch. At this time, the infant should play with toys that he can shake, bang, or pull. He will also enjoy playing "peek-a-boo."

By age 8 months to 1 year, the infant uses his abilities as a stepping stone to learn new skills. He can remove an obstacle blocking his way to an object or goal. He also attempts to climb and to push away. At this stage of development, encourage caregivers to praise the child's achievements verbally and to check his environment for safety. In the hospital, provide a canopy on the crib.

Language. Crying is the infant's first vocalization. At age 5 to 6 weeks, he is capable of making small, throaty sounds. At age 3 to 4 months, he gurgles and laughs aloud. By age 8 months, he usually can make vowel and consonant sounds. By age 9 or 10 months, he usually understands the word "no" and responds to his name. By age 1 year, he usually associates meaning to sound.

When caring for the infant in the hospital, keep in mind the following points:
• Remember to talk to him and to smile and laugh when giving care.
• Use the correct pronunciation of words, not baby talk.
• Call the infant by the same name his caregivers use.
• Avoid overusing the word "no." Limit its need by adapting the child's environment to eliminate temptations.

Nursing considerations

Medication. Because of his developing motor ability, an infant is capable of resisting medication. When administering medication, hold the infant firmly in a comforting, not punitive, manner. During the later stages of infancy, the infant will be learning to drink from a cup. Be prepared for spitting. A small cup or syringe is usually more effective and less likely to cause spitting than using a spoon.

Keep in mind that the infant is capable of remembering negative experiences. To prevent future negative responses to medication administration, be sure to provide physical and verbal comfort measures.

Nutrition. During the first 6 months, human milk is the most desirable form of nutrition. However, commercially prepared infant formulas are an appropriate alternative (see *Common nutritional sources for infants,* page 4.)

Solid foods should be introduced into the diet by age 5 or 6 months. Before that time, solid foods are incompatible with the infant's GI functioning; the GI system may be exposed to food antigens, which could provoke allergy. Avoid pushing or forcing solid foods on the infant. Loss of the extrusion reflex (usually by age 4 or 5 months) indicates his readiness for solid foods.

When introducing solid foods, use rice cereal, preferably a commercially prepared infant cereal. Such cereals are easily digested and are associated with a low allergic reaction. Mix the cereal with formula (mix it with juice for breast-fed infants). Remember to feed the infant solid foods with a spoon, never from a bottle.

From age 7 months to 1 year, the infant still depends on human milk or formula as his primary source of nutrition; during this time, new foods should be introduced one at a time. The usual progression is cereal, followed by fruit, then vegetables, then meat. If using jarred foods, be sure to store opened jars in the refrigerator. Never feed the infant directly from a jar; instead, use a clean bowl and spoon to avoid introducing bacteria into the jar. When he is able to sit, feed him the solid portion of his meal while he is positioned in a high chair.

At age 9 months to 1 year, the infant will be drinking a small amount of liquid from a cup or glass with assistance. At this time, he should be held while he is finishing milk from a bottle. Infants who are held when nippling usually sense warmth and security and wean more easily. Encourage self-help in feeding. The infant's sense of independence is developing at this time. He should begin advancing from finger foods to holding a spoon.

Safety considerations. An infant tends to wiggle and squirm and may cross a wide expanse of territory. Remember to always keep one hand on the infant whenever the crib rail is down or the Isolette is open. Also, keep in mind that the gap between the mattress and side of the crib is dangerous. Fill any gaps with a blanket roll.

Other safety considerations include the following:
• Do not prop up a bottle to feed the infant or position him on his back after feeding because he may regurgitate and aspirate. Also, avoid feeding him nuts, corn, unpeeled hot dogs, and pills or tablets.
• Inspect all toys for sharp edges and loose parts.
• When carrying the infant, protect his head by shielding it with your hand. (Infants are extremely vulnerable to injury from dropping, bumping, and falling.)
• Keep all harmful objects out of the infant's reach. (Infants explore objects with their mouths.)
• Never leave an infant alone in a tub unattended; he is helpless in water.
• When the infant can stand, remove crib bumpers and use a crib canopy; standing indicates a readiness to climb. Keep in mind that the infant may be stimulated to climb and explore because of the unfamiliar hospital environment.

Participation of the primary caregiver. When the infant is hospitalized, allow unrestricted visiting, thereby encouraging the caregiver to stay with him and to assist with his care. However, keep in mind that the caregiver's anxiety, frustration, and fear may stimulate the child to exhibit negative behavior. Remain at the child's bedside to provide physical and emotional support.

Toddler period
The toddler period extends from age 1 to 3.

Physical characteristics

Growth. During the toddler years, the child's growth slows; however, his strength and motor skills increase. Weight gain is approximately 5 lb (2.3 kg) per year; by age 30 months, the child normally weighs four times his birth weight (see "Physical Growth Charts" in the Appendices). Most body systems will have reached physiologic maturity by the end of the toddler period.

Although the child's height at this time increases about 3″ (7.6 cm) per year, the growth occurs in uneven spurts rather than uniformly and consistently. A male child's adult height can be estimated by doubling his height at age 2; a female child's adult height, by doubling her height at age 18 months.

Head. Head circumference measurements continue to be important during the toddler years. Usually, the circumference increases 1″ (2.5 cm) between ages 1 and 2 and is equal to the chest circumference.

Chest. By age 3, the chest circumference is greater than the head circumference.

Skin. Unlike an infant's skin, which is thin and delicate, the toddler's dermis and epidermis are bonded for improved barrier protection against infection. This bonding also makes the skin less fragile, improving the ease of skin care.

Motor development. The toddler years are a period of intense activity and exploration. The child develops greater purposeful mobility, such as running and climbing. During this time, advise caregivers to avoid clothing the child in restrictive garments and to be aware of safety concerns.

Temperature. The toddler's body temperature is more stable because of improved physiologic control through shivering and capillary constriction and dilation. Also, the child can control his temperature because of his greater motor ability, which allows him to put on or take off clothing.

Sleep pattern. You will note wide individual differences in sleep patterns during the toddler years. A child age 1 to 2 usually takes two naps during the day, whereas a child age 3 only takes one nap per day. Usually, toddlers sleep through the night, approximately 9 to 12 hours. Nightmares or night terrors commonly begin at age 2 to 3.

When caring for the toddler in the hospital, try to arrange naps according to the child's home schedule. Also, plan interventions to avoid interrupting his sleep. Provide quiet comfort and reassurance when nightmares occur.

Try to find out about the child's home rituals for bedtime; stories and singing may help prepare him for sleep. If the child usually finds comfort in a transitional object, such as a soft blanket or cuddly toy, do not attempt to wash or alter the object in any way during his hospitalization; this could destroy its comforting familiarity. Also, avoid placing too many toys in his crib; this may stimulate him and keep him awake.

Elimination. Toddlers are at an age of toilet readiness; myelination of the spinal cord permits sphincter control. Bowel control and daytime bladder control are usually achieved by age 3. At this time, the toddler's bladder capacity increases, and the kidneys are better able to concentrate urine.

When caring for the toddler in the hospital, be sure to inquire on admission whether he is toilet trained. Also ask what words he associates with toileting and whether he is on a regular schedule. Be consistent with home routines; however, be aware that his toileting habits may regress during hospitalization because of stress.

Fecal smearing is not unusual with a child age 15 to 20 months. If the toddler engages in fecal smearing, be sure to fasten his diapers securely, changing them immediately after each bowel movement. Prepare caregivers for the possiblity of fecal smearing. Encourage them to help channel the child's impulse to smear by introducing him to finger painting and working with clay.

Psychosocial characteristics

According to Erikson's theory, the toddler period (stage II) focuses on autonomy (self-control and will power) versus shame and doubt. Temper tantrums, negativism, and disciplinary problems are the hallmarks of this age-group as the child learns to control his environment and express his will. He wants to do things for himself, demands immediate gratification, and manifests rapid mood changes.

According to Freud, toddlers are egocentric and possessive and struggle with holding-on and letting-go behaviors (anal stage). Toddlers usually begin to imitate sex role behavior. Toys are the focus of play because interaction with other children is minimal (parallel play).

During this stage of development, the child should be permitted as much freedom and opportunity for self-care as is safe and reasonable; forced dependence will produce self-doubt. Encourage caregivers to dress the child in clothing he can manage independently.

Discipline during this stage should be a demonstration of love, not anger. The toddler needs limits set on unacceptable demands; such limits offer security. He should be praised liberally, but only when deserved.

Hospitalization threatens the toddler's sense of security and autonomy and may result in regression (marked by loss of acquired skills, temper tantrums, or unusual passivity). Keep in mind that he is at an age when he fears strangers; however, the older the toddler, the better he will tolerate separation from his caregivers. Usually, a toddler responds better to staff members when a caregiver is present.

Other nursing tips to keep in mind include the following:

• Remember to use regular patterns in all aspects of your care to promote the child's independence and sense of security, especially if he is passive.

• Approach the child slowly in a nonthreatening manner, greeting him from a distance.

• Make sure that you work with other staff members to promote a consistent nurse-patient relationship with the child.

Cognition. According to Piaget's theory, the sensorimotor stage extends to approximately age 2. The child then enters the preoperational stage, in which he begins using a trial-and-error method of thinking and reasoning. The child develops object permanence, the realization that objects beyond his immediate view still exist.

Because the toddler's sense of time is beginning to develop, he usually can "wait a minute"; however, avoid long waits whenever possible.

The toddler thinks in terms of magical or omnipotent thought processes: he believes he can simply wish for something to happen. Guilt may develop because he blames himself for any untoward happenings.

During this stage, caregivers must watch their actions and words because the toddler will imitate them. Provide the child with opportunities for positive imitative play, such as with toy telephones, dolls, and toy workshop and household tools.

Speech and language. Development in this area is usually rapid, with girls developing faster than boys. However, such development may be slowed or arrested by trauma or illness. Keep this in mind when explaining procedures to the child. Be sure to explain all procedures as simply as possible. Play techniques will help him to gain understanding through participation.

The toddler's comprehension usually exceeds his capacity for speech. Only about one third of his speech is intelligible. The number of words used in an average response approximately equals the child's age in years. He uses his favorite word, "no," to exercise autonomy.

Toddlers enjoy simple songs with repetitive rhymes as well as moving in time to music. A musical activity should be scheduled into each day.

Animism. The toddler treats objects as if they are alive (for example, if a child falls, he may spank the floor for hurting him). He assumes that things occur because of cause and effect, especially when events are closely related in time. At about age 12 to 18 months, he begins to realize the relationship of one object to another. At this time, he should be introduced to nested toys, toys with parts that open and close, and toys designed for pounding, such as hammers and drums.

Memory. The toddler's memory is developing at this time. Because he associates painful experiences with specific settings and people, you'll need to prepare him with an honest, adequate explanation before any procedure. His attention span, although short, is improving. For example, a child age 16 months usually can remain at one task, such as looking at books or playing with blocks, for approximately 10 minutes; a child age 24 months can remain at a set task for 15 to 30 minutes and can put on his own pants, shoes, and socks. Toddlers should be exposed to various toys and activities frequently.

Nursing considerations

Medication. To foster the toddler's developing sense of autonomy, you'll need to give him a certain amount of freedom in choosing how to take his medication. Provide acceptable choices, such as which drink he can take with his medication and where he can sit when taking it; however, avoid mentioning choices when no choice is possible. If chewable medication is available, you might allow him to choose between chewable tablets and the liquid form.

The toddler prefers to sit or stand (rather than lie down) when taking oral medications. He may spit out the medication deliberately; this is a manifestation of negativism, common for this age-group. When giving medication, have the toddler sit in a chair or on your lap. Avoid holding him down; hold him only to support him and to offer comfort. Ask his caregivers what methods work best at home.

Because the toddler will resist swallowing anything that tastes bad, mix medication in a small amount of applesauce, pudding, or other soft food (after first checking for compatibility). However, avoid associating medication with an essential food. When administering the medication, be firm and consistent, but also be kind and honest. For instance, explain that you are giving him medication mixed in applesauce because it will help make it taste better. Also, tell him that the taste will last only a minute.

When giving medication by I.M. injection, the vastus lateralis—the largest muscle mass in children under age 3—is the preferred injection site because it avoids blood vessels and nerves.

Keep in mind that toddlers are easily distracted. When giving an injection, try distracting the child by talking to him, letting him play with a toy, or having him look at pictures. Also keep in mind that he may cry when injected. Give him permission to cry, then comfort him. Never lie about potential pain.

Also remember that a child in this age-group has good motor control that permits grabbing and throwing. Be sure to keep the medication tray or cart well out of his reach.

Nutrition. Because the toddler years are important for developing good eating habits, avoid using food as a reward or punishment. Children in this age-group require approximately 45 calories per lb (100 calories per kg) of body weight each day; caloric intake must be sufficient for growth, healing, and energy.

Milk intake should not exceed 2 or 3 cups per day. Weaning should occur at about age 1. Snacks should provide quality nutrition; nonnutritional fats and sweets should be avoided.

The toddler's stomach capacity increases from about 200 ml at age 1 to greater than 500 ml at age 3. During this period, the child's GI tract has developed into a more advanced state with a slowed transit time from the stomach to the anus. Usually, a toddler should be fed three meals a day; however, if the child has a fever, his basal metabolic needs will increase and he'll require more frequent meals. The toddler's fluid requirements, normally about 2 oz per lb of body weight per day, will increase by about 10% with each degree of fever.

The toddler's sense of taste is not yet refined; plain foods are best. Usually, he will eat only one food at a time. Also, the toddler's appetite should be expected to fluctuate (between pickiness and binges) according to his individual growth spurts and plateaus. This is known as *physiologic anorexia*. Reassure caregivers that this is normal, and tell them never to force the child to eat, but rather to provide smaller portions.

Note the following additional nutritional considerations:
• Encourage the toddler's development of autonomy. Remember that at age 15 months, he can drink from a cup with little or no spilling, and at age 18 months, he can use a spoon to feed himself for adequate nutritional intake. Be sure to cut his food into small pieces for self-feeding and to provide a cup and spoon.
• Do not expect neatness or scold him if he makes a mess. Remember to make mealtimes happy times.
• Keep in mind that the toddler may refuse to eat as a means of controlling the situation, especially if he senses adult concern.
• Because the toddler's sense of security is based on ritual and routine, plan for regular times and places for meals, if possible.
• Because the toddler does not mind repetition of his diet and hesitates to try new foods, obtain a list of his likes and dislikes from his caregivers. To avoid causing stress, use the same dish, cup, and spoon for each meal.

Safety considerations. Because more toddlers die or become disabled from accidents than from any other cause, an important part of the nurse's responsibility involves teaching safety guidelines and accident prevention. Children age 2 to 3 are at greatest risk for accidents. Although still clumsy, they can move (by walking, running, or climbing) toward any object they are determined to reach and have little awareness of danger.

Common injuries include falls, burns, and collisions (with animate or inanimate objects). Most accidents occur in or near the home during a child's exploration of motor skills. Poisoning commonly occurs in toddlers because of their inability to discriminate tastes.

When providing safety guidelines to caregivers, keep in mind the following points:
• Stress the need to be careful of what the child is carrying when walking. Also point out the danger of toys with sharp edges.
• Explain that a definite correlation exists between personality type and proneness to accidents. Tell them to be alert if the child exhibits active "daredevil-like" behavioral tendencies.
• Encourage them to provide the child with washable toys without small removable parts. Ask them to bring the child a few favorite toys from home; be sure to check them for safety.

Participation of the primary caregiver. When a toddler is hospitalized, unlimited visiting or rooming-in is desirable to minimize emotional distress resulting from the child's separation from his caregivers. Make sure that comfortable chairs and cots are provided, as needed. Also, be sure to order meals for the caregivers or to relieve them for meals.

Advise the caregivers to tell the toddler when they are leaving the room to prevent feelings of mistrust resulting from their "sneaking out." Explain that temper tantrums may result if the child feels insecure because of their frequent absence.

Explain that children express separation anxiety in three stages: protest, despair, and denial. Depending on the toddler's anxiety stage, he may show no emotion whatsoever when the caregivers return. Reassure the caregivers that the deeper and more emotionally traumatic levels of anxiety may be prevented by visiting at least once during every 24-hour period.

Consistency in care demands careful adherence to the nursing care plan. This care plan must include essential information from the primary caregiver. Be sure to ask about the child's routines and rituals, and try to enlist help in the child's daily care. Because the caregiver's role as the child's comforter is important, provide frequent opportunities for hugging after injections and other procedures.

Be aware that the primary caregiver needs to feel useful and needed and that the toddler will quickly perceive any anxiety concerning these needs. Continually ask for input concerning the child's personality, likes and dislikes, and idiosyncrasies. Also, assess the caregiver's desire and ability to be present during procedures and activities. Rarely, caregivers do not wish to be present. Offer assurance that this is all right. Your concern and interest will be appreciated.

Preschool period
The preschool years extend from age 3 to 6.

Physical characteristics

Growth. During the preschool years, the child's growth stabilizes. He usually gains approximately 5 lb (2.3 kg) per year and doubles his birth weight by age 4 or 5. Height usually increases by 2½" to 3" (6.4 to 7.6 cm) per year.

Sleep pattern. The preschooler's sleeping pattern is well established by this time. However, he may develop a fear of the dark, ghosts, or monsters. When hospitalized, the preschooler should be maintained on his routine home sleeping schedule. Provide him with transitional objects, such as a soft toy or blanket, and soft lighting. Discuss any of his fears openly with him.

Elimination. By age 3, the child usually has established diurnal control of his bowel and bladder. Nocturnal control is usually achieved by age 4½. Hospitalization, however, may result in regression of his elimination patterns. To avoid making him feel guilty, refer to any regression as an accident. As appropriate, provide him with opportunities to assume responsibility for any accidents (for instance, allow him to help change the sheets).

Psychosocial characteristics

According to Erikson's theory, the preschool stage (stage III) is one of initiative versus guilt (in which the child wants to learn what he can do for himself). The child wants to please others and usually will cooperate with procedures; however, he may perceive any pain or restraint associated with a procedure as a punishment. Role-playing with honest explanations can help prepare the child for procedures.

The preschooler usually tolerates separation from his caregivers without any great stress. When caring for the preschooler in the hospital, try to learn the names of his siblings, pets, and friends and refer to them often. He may exhibit a vivid imagination and even talk to imaginary friends. Acknowledge his imaginary friends, but refer to them as being imaginary, not real.

Other considerations to keep in mind when caring for the preschooler in the hospital are as follows:
• As part of his independent nature, the preschooler will want to dress and care for himself. Make a point of praising his efforts, and allow him to make acceptable choices (for example, ask him if he wants to wear his red or blue pants to physical therapy, *not* whether he wants to go to physical therapy).
• Preschoolers typically enjoy repetitive, interactive, formal-type games. If your preschool-age patient is ambulatory, encourage him to play "London Bridge," "Ring-Around-A-Rosy," "Simon Says," or similar games.
• The preschooler may try to perform beyond his abilities and feel guilty if he fails to achieve his goals. Structure activities to ensure his success (for example, give him puzzles that are not too difficult).

• Because the preschooler is at an age when he is developing a conscience and a sense of morality, establish rules and limits on his behavior.

Cognition. According to Piaget's theory, the preschool years are when a child develops concrete thinking; learning depends primarily on the senses. In the hospital, he should be allowed to see, hear, and feel any medical equipment and should receive honest answers to his questions and appropriate demonstrations on a doll or toy animal. (The preschooler's favorite word is "why" and he will persist relentlessly in asking "why" questions until he receives answers.)

The preschooler generally takes things literally. Keep in mind that, in the hospital, a preschool-age patient may interpret the word "dye" to mean "die" when he hears discussions about X-ray examinations.

The preschooler understands time best in terms of daily activities. Therefore, refer to anticipated events in terms of "after lunch" or "before bedtime" or in relation to other routine activities. Also, because he believes that his thoughts cause events to occur, reassure him that any problems and unhappy events do not result from his naughty thoughts.

The preschool years are also a time for normal sexual curiosity and exploration. Masturbation is not uncommon among preschoolers. To avoid overreaction, reassure caregivers that this is normal.

Speech and language. A preschooler's vocabulary typically expands from approximately 900 words at age 3 to over 2,000 words at age 5. Rhymes, songs, and exercises in cadence can be used to elicit his interest and cooperation.

Although the preschooler uses sentences well, he may stutter or hesitate when speaking. Advise caregivers to ignore any stuttering or hesitation at this time. The preschooler is capable of following simple commands; however, he shouldn't be given a number of commands at one time.

Nursing considerations

Medication. When giving medication to a preschooler, keep in mind the following points:
• Because the preschooler may believe that his "insides" will ooze out through a needle puncture site, always provide an adhesive bandage to "seal the hole."
• A preschooler's thoughts are generally centered on one aspect of an object or situation at a time (for example, he will focus on the height or width of a medicine glass, but not on both simultaneously). When he refuses to take a medication, try offering it again in a different container.
• He may prefer chewable tablets to the liquid form of a medica-

tion; ask him which form he would prefer, if both are available. Also, avoid calling medication candy and never lie about the taste.

• If the child has been walking for more than a year, his gluteal muscles are probably developed enough for receiving I.M. injections. If the muscle is well developed, the gluteal site may be used in addition to the vastus lateralis site.

• Although not fully developed until adolescence, the deltoid muscle may be used with extreme caution for I.M. injection of medications that require rapid absorption. The muscle is small and close to the radial nerve. More rapid absorption occurs because of the muscle's proximity to a better blood supply than other I.M. sites.

• Because the preschooler may expect an immediate cure, explain to him, in appropriate terms, that the medication will take time to travel to the "sick part," but that it will help.

Nutrition. A preschool-age child requires approximately 40 calories per lb (about 90 calories per kg) of body weight per day. About 15% of his diet should be supplied as protein.

A preschooler can feed himself completely and often resents any assistance. Because he enjoys a wide variety of foods, make a point of learning his food preferences, including ethnic variations, and offer him appropriate choices. Also, experiment with various sizes and shapes of plates, cups, and utensils to determine his preference.

Safety considerations. Better coordinated and less accident-prone than a toddler, a preschooler can reason with an adult and requires fewer safety barriers. A child age 3 requires close supervision, whereas a child age 4 to 5 is more aware of dangerous situations and can avoid potential hazards when they are pointed out to him.

Participation of the primary caregiver. Encourage the caregiver to room-in with the hospitalized child. If this is impossible, caregivers should establish a consistent and predictable visiting schedule. Advise the primary caregiver to be truthful with the child about absences and to prepare him for times of separation.

Encourage the caregiver to participate in the child's play activities and to provide and care for any nonhospital clothing (such clothing focuses on the child's wellness rather than illness).

The caregiver may also help with nurturing the child when he is unable to care for himself and with preparing him for procedures. When eliciting the caregiver's help in these areas, be sure to prepare the caregiver and to offer assistance. Avoid using medical terms when explaining procedures. Encourage the caregiver to support and comfort the child during and after painful procedures; however, don't ask the caregiver to restrain the child or to participate in any painful procedure.

Middle childhood period

The middle childhood years extend from age 6 to 11.

Physical characteristics

Growth. Typically, the middle childhood years are ones of gradual, steady, even progress in physical and emotional growth. Between ages 6 and 12, the child's height normally increases 1″ to 2″ (2.5 to 5 cm) per year and his weight 3 to 6 lb (1.4 to 2.7 kg) per year. Changes in body proportion are marked by development of a longer hip line and gradual loss of body fat.

Teeth. During this age, the child's deciduous teeth are replaced with permanent teeth. Remember to check for any loose teeth before administering an anesthetic, as an unconscious child may swallow or aspirate a dislodged tooth.

Maturation of body systems. The child's GI system develops to withstand an increased capacity, resulting in fewer stomach upsets. His bladder capacity also increases. Pulse and respiratory rates generally decrease and blood pressure increases (see *Taking a child's blood pressure,* and *Vital sign measurements,* page 23).

Because bone mineralization is incomplete at this time, the child should avoid injury to bones and muscles; trauma in these areas may alter growth.

Activity and muscle coordination. The child in this age-group needs regular exercise to promote muscle coordination of his developing capacities. As his fine muscle coordination improves, he may develop artistic outlets, such as playing a musical instrument, as a form of self-expression.

Physical maturation. Wide differences, especially in terms of developmental rate, are noted among all children of this age-group; however, the greatest discrepancies occur between the sexes. Girls tend to develop faster than boys, typically reaching puberty 2 years earlier. A child who perceives himself negatively as being different from his peers may need reassurance that his uniqueness is a normal part of growing up.

Psychosocial characteristics

During the middle childhood years, the child's unique personality characteristics emerge. He is able to assume increasing responsibilities in meeting personal needs. According to Erikson's theory, a child in this age-group struggles with industry versus inferiority. At a stage when he enjoys personal accomplishment, he is eager to build on his own skills to become a useful, productive person, which serves to strengthen his self-concept. During this stage, he needs reinforcement of his accomplishments to develop a sense of adequacy.

At this age, the child is motivated intrinsically by independent

TAKING A CHILD'S BLOOD PRESSURE

Taking a child's blood pressure may be easier said than done, especially if he's anxious and uncooperative. Read what follows for some tips to make the task easier—for you *and* your patient.

Encouraging cooperation

For best results, always try to take blood pressure readings when your patient's calm and relaxed. But a pediatric patient may not be so accommodating. You may have to contend with a child who's restless, anxious, or combative. Take time to establish rapport with the child and gain his confidence. Show him the blood pressure equipment; then, take his caretaker's blood pressure to show him that the procedure won't hurt. If he seems uncomfortable or frightened by lying on the examining table, allow him to sit up.

Taking readings

A child's blood pressure fluctuates more than an adult's. So, to get an accurate blood pressure measurement, you'll need to take at least three readings at different times.

Some controversy exists over which Korotkoff phase to document as the diastolic measurement—the muffled 4th phase, which may provide a false-high reading, or the hard-to-detect 5th phase, which may provide a false-low reading. The best you can do is to document both phases; for example, 130/76/62 (I/IV/V).

Note: When taking a reading, don't press the stethoscope's diaphragm too hard against the antecubital fossa. You may distort the Korotkoff sounds.

Selecting the proper blood pressure cuff

Which cuff size is appropriate for your pediatric patient? Use the following chart as a guide.

Important: If your patient's unusually large or small for his age group, select a cuff that's appropriate for his *size,* not his age.

Age category	Cuff width	Cuff length
Newborn	2.5 to 4 cm	5 to 10 cm
Infant	6 to 8 cm	12 to 13.5 cm
Child	9 to 10 cm	17 to 22.5 cm
Adult	12 to 13 cm	22 to 23.5 cm

Selecting the proper blood pressure method

In addition to determining cuff size, your pediatric patient's age and size influence the method you use to take his blood pressure. Choose from among the three noninvasive alternatives.

The ultrasound method

When examining a newborn (either premature or full-term), use an ultrasound Doppler monitor. More accurate than the sphygmomanometer, the ultrasound monitor picks up frequency changes produced by blood flow variations and either amplifies the sounds or represents them on an oscilloscope. This gives you an accurate systolic pressure reading and a good estimate of diastolic pressure in most infants.

The flush method

When examining an infant less than age 1, use the flush method if the Doppler monitor isn't available. Here's how:
• Apply a proper-size blood pressure cuff.
• Elevate the infant's arm or thigh (either will do because the arm and thigh pressures of a child this age are equal).
• Wrap an elastic bandage from his wrist to his elbow or from his ankle to his knee.
• Wait until his hand (or foot) becomes pale; then, inflate the blood pressure cuff.
• Unwrap the bandage, and begin deflating the cuff. Note the pressure reading when the hand or foot flushes from blood return.

This approximate reading isn't the infant's systolic or diastolic pressure, but rather his mean arterial blood pressure. In infants this age, the upper limit of normal flush pressure is approximately 80 mm Hg.

Conventional method

When examining a child who's age 3 or older, use a conventional blood pressure cuff and sphygmomanometer. Because a child's Korotkoff sounds are harder to hear than an adult's, remember to take the reading in a quiet setting.

Source: *Report of the Task Force on Blood Pressure Control in Children,* The National Heart, Lung, and Blood Institute (NHLBI), 1977

behavior to control his environment and gain the approval of his peers. Peer relationships provide opportunities for learning to handle feelings of hostility and to interact with others in positions of authority and leadership. A child with chronic health problems usually will respond well in self-help group settings at this stage.

Extrinsically motivated by material rewards and the need for recognition, the child wants to succeed. Use rewards at this time to encourage compliance with treatment and care.

Cognition. According to Piaget's theory, during the middle childhood years, the child focuses on concrete operations because he is able to verbalize actions or processes and to perform such operations mentally. He generally becomes more flexible in conceptualization and seeing things from other perspectives, and he progresses in making judgments through reasoning. At this age, the child will respond well to teaching on health maintenance and preventing illness.

Moral development. At age 6 to 7, the child usually interprets and judges an action by its consequences. For instance, he may interpret an accident or illness as punishment for previous misdeeds. The older child (age 8 to 10), who is beginning to develop reasoning, interprets events as less absolute. He is better able to understand the needs and desires of others.

Play. Children in this age-group can participate in quiet games and activities and follow rules. Working on collections, playing board and card games, and reading (or being read to) are good diversions for a hospitalized child.

Imagination of an event may stimulate the child's ability to feel in control of the situation. Threatening events, such as difficult hospital procedures, can be preceded with a play activity that allows the child to imagine he has gained control over the event or situation.

Nursing considerations

Medication. When administering medication, always tell the child why he is receiving the medication. The child's understanding improves his cooperation and compliance with the regimen.

Also, allow him to choose the form of medication (tablets or liquid) as well as the time schedule, as allowed. This fosters his sense of being in control. If at all possible, cooperate with the child in developing his acceptance of threatening or painful procedures or events rather than trying to force him to comply with doctor's orders.

Sleep pattern. A child in this age-group usually requires no nap time. By age 6, he usually sleeps about 11 to 12 hours a night; by age 10, about 9 to 10 hours a night. If allowed to stay up later at night, the child may feel fatigued the next day. Although the child may be able to give several reasons for resisting bedtime, a

VITAL SIGN MEASUREMENTS

Age	Temperature	Pulse rate	Respiratory rate	Blood pressure
Under 1 year	99.1° F.* (37.3° C.)	80 to 160/minute (Newborn: 70 to 170/minute)	20 to 40/minute (Newborn: 30 to 80/minute)	63 mm Hg mean (using flush technique)
2 years	98.8° to 99.1° F. (37.1° to 37.3° C.)	80 to 120/minute	24 to 25/minute	96/30 mm Hg
4 years	98.5° to 98.9° F. (36.9° to 37.2° C.)	80 to 120/minute	22 to 24/minute	98/60 mm Hg
6 years	98.4° to 98.5° F. (36.9° C.)	75 to 115/minute	21 to 22/minute	105/60 mm Hg
10 years	98.0° to 98.2° F. (36.7° to 36.8° C.)	70 to 110/minute	19/minute	112/64 mm Hg
14 years	97.6° to 97.9° F. (36.4° to 36.6° C.)	65 to 100/minute	18/minute	120/75 mm Hg

*Rectal temperature

strict lights-out policy on the unit should ensure compliance with bedtime rules.

Nutrition. During middle childhood, a child requires a balanced diet for optimal growth. Use mealtimes and other events to teach the importance of adequate nutritional intake.

At this stage of development, the child will be acquiring a taste for an increasing variety of foods. Stimulate his appetite by allowing choices of foods, when appropriate. Keep in mind, however, that most children enjoy junk food. Allow him to choose such foods if they have adequate nutritional value and are allowed in his dietary regimen.

Safety considerations. Because a child of this age-group has refined muscle coordination and can determine on his own when safety is threatened, he is less prone to accidents. Keep in mind, however, that a hospitalized child is usually stressed and therefore more susceptible to accidents. Caution him to use extra care.

Sex education. Children in this age-group should be prepared for prepubertal changes (puberty in girls may occur as early as age 8). Children should recognize sexual differences (that is, in the development of secondary sex characteristics and of physical strength and endurance). Reinforce each child's sense of adequacy and accomplishment.

Participation of the primary caregiver. Remember to include the child's family in all health care teaching. During this stage of the child's development, family members remain the greatest influence on the child's developing personality. They set behavioral standards and are the basis for the child's value system.

The child also needs the security of an authority figure. Although caregivers may release some of their control to the child's peer relationships, they still need to help establish and maintain control over the child's impulsive behavior.

Because children typically regress to a more dependent status when sick or hospitalized, encourage the caregiver to remain at the child's bedside or to contact him frequently by telephone.

Because children imitate adults, encourage the caregivers to set a positive example for the child by demonstrating desirable behavior in response to threatening or traumatic events (such as hospital procedures and surgery).

Prepubertal period
The prepubertal period extends from age 11 to 13.

Physical characteristics
Growth and development. The prepubertal period is one of rapid growth and developmental change. A prepubertal growth spurt typically occurs earlier in girls; strength and endurance are usually greater in boys.

Girls normally experience a height increase of 5½" to 6" (14 to 15.2 cm). Subcutaneous fat is deposited in their chest, hips, arms, and calves. Body contours change (for example, the hips broaden).

Girls, as a group, demonstrate a wide variance in individual shape and size, whereas boys tend to appear more uniform as a group. During this period, boys sometimes experience transient obesity, which is later replaced by bone and muscle mass. Shoulders broaden. Height does not increase as early in boys. (During this period, a boy usually attains 80% of his adult height.)

Glandular development. At this stage of development, boys and girls tend to blush easily because of vasomotor instability. They also have active sebaceous glands and increased perspiration from glandular activity. Capable of understanding the importance of good hygiene, they should be instructed about the use of deodorants.

Energy level and self-care. The prepubertal child can be helpful to a much younger child; however, he may show sibling rivalry if the younger child is relatively close to his age. He is capable of and prefers self-care; consider this when developing the nursing care plan.

Often energetic and enthusiastic, he may manifest pent-up energy by fidgeting or drumming his fingers. Depending on his health status, provide him with appropriate outlets for his energy, such as a punching ball, musical instrument, or stationary bike.

Sleep pattern. Because the prepubertal child will stay up late if permitted to do so, be sure to establish rules and limitations in the hospital setting. Requiring 9 to 10 hours of sleep a night, he tends to arouse more easily in the morning than when younger.

Elimination. By this age, the child has well-established elimination patterns; persistent enuresis usually resolves around this time. Very much aware of body changes, he usually demands privacy and does not readily discuss elimination.

Psychosocial characteristics

According to Erikson's theory, the prepubertal period is a transitional phase between periods of industry versus inferiority (middle childhood) and identity versus role confusion (adolescence). The prepubertal child is often introspective and self-critical, comparing himself with an idealized self-image. He needs assistance with ego-strengthening efforts while learning to repect the rights and opinions of others. If placed in a hospital room or an area with younger children, he will resent being on the "baby floor."

Because a child in this age-group typically is interested in learning about his body and health-related matters, provide him with information about his admission diagnosis.

Preoccupied with appearance (particularly with hair and clothes) but not necessarily with hygiene, the prepubertal child takes a long time to prepare himself for visitors or procedures. Be sure to allow him sufficient time to prepare for procedures; however, keep in mind that you may need to remind him to bathe and brush his teeth.

Vacillating between dependence and independence, the prepubertal child may rebel against adult standards as an expression of independence. He may resort to arguing. The prepubertal child may begin smoking as a demonstration of rebellion or an attempt to look mature.

The prepubertal child may select an adult outside of his immediate family to imitate, identify with, or fantasize about (hero worship). He may even develop a crush on an adult (sometimes the nurse).

Interpersonal relationships within this age group are sources of anxiety and stress. The prepubertal child seeks peer group acceptance and will try to conform. He often confides in his peers rather than family members and enjoys group activities involving his peers. At this time, he begins to desire a relationship with the opposite sex. Adults must prepare for questions during this period of discovery.

Body changes resulting from illness or trauma are a major threat to the child's self-esteem. When caring for a child with such body changes, remember to exercise extreme caution with your body language and facial expressions in response to his altered appearance.

Because brooding and withdrawal are the prepubertal child's usual means of expressing frustration, he should be allowed privacy until he is ready to talk. He is capable of exercising great self-control when in physical pain and usually will not resist painful procedures; however, although he appears in control, he needs preparation and comforting.

Cognition. According to Piaget's theory, the prepubertal child is in a transitional state from concrete to formal operational thought patterns. He is beginning to use logic and to show consistency in decision-making and problem-solving abilities. Never assume, however, that the child is completely into the formal operational stage; be available to listen and offer explanations.

Nursing considerations

Medication. When administering medications to prepubertal children, be extremely careful to check all patient identifications first. Although usually cooperative, children of this age-group enjoy playing practical jokes, such as switching beds or answering to another child's name when called; however, they are not always aware of the potential danger of playing such jokes.

Nutrition. Prepubertal boys generally require 2,800 calories per day; girls, approximately 2,400 calories per day. For both sexes, at least 15% of these calories should be supplied as protein.

Keep in mind that snacks may be the mainstay of the child's diet and that junk foods and fad-type foods are typically preferred at this age. To help ensure that the child meets his caloric requirements, try incorporating nutritious junk foods high in calcium and iron, such as pizza and cheeseburgers, into his diet.

Prepubescence is a crucial time (sometimes a turning point) for weight problems in many children. Obese children may have a weight problem for life. Girls may begin worrying about their weight even when no problem exists. Be alert to the danger signs of eating disorders. Use role models when appropriate, and offer guidance and advice without preaching.

Safety considerations. Children in this age-group are often prone to take a dare or attempt a feat to gain peer acceptance or save face. Promote the child's self-esteem to reduce his need for seeking status in dangerous ways.

Other considerations to keep in mind include the following:
• Because hospitalized children may roughhouse if feeling well enough, provide supervised outlets for excess energy.
• Sometimes children have accidents to gain attention. They may be reacting to a situation or expressing anger. To help reduce the likelihood of this accident potential, pay attention to the child's positive behaviors and explore the cause of anger.

Participation of the primary caregiver. Because family support is essential to the prepubertal child, advise caregivers to offer consistent and caring support. Although the child doesn't require their continued presence, he does need to know that their support is available.

The child may not appreciate the caregiver's open demonstrations of affection and may even display better manners and cooperation when the caregiver is not present. Try to arrive at a compromise on the amount of time the caregiver will spend visiting the child in the hospital.

The caregiver may be frustrated by constant arguments with the child. Be supportive and explain that this does not indicate a lack of love. Help the caregiver to understand that the prepubertal period is a difficult stage and that the child's feelings of antagonism or guilt are typical.

Adolescent period

Adolescence extends from age 13 to 18.

Physical characteristics

Growth and development. By the time a child reaches adolescence, his individual growth pattern is well established. He has increased speed, coordination, and strength. By age 15, secondary sex characteristics usually have developed fully. Adult facial features and stature usually develop by about age 18 in girls and age 20 in boys.

During adolescence, the legs lengthen and shoulders broaden in boys. In girls, fat accumulates in the shoulders, hips, breasts, and thighs. Menstrual periods usually occur regularly. Bone density increases, and muscle represents a larger percentage of body weight.

Sleep pattern. By adolescence, patterns of work, school, and sleep generally are well established—except on weekends, when the child may stay up late, then sleep longer to catch up on lost sleep.

Elimination. Elimination patterns are well established by adolescence. Although the adolescent is capable of recognizing the usual quality of his own urine and feces, he may need information about normal body functioning. Encourage him to report any unusual signs and symptoms.

Psychosocial characteristics

According to Erikson's theory, adolescence typically is characterized by identity versus role confusion (in which the child is striving to become more independent, vacillating between independent and dependent roles). The adolescent commonly has mood swings.

He may rebel against restrictions and rules and may be frequently absent from home as his activities become more peer-centered rather than family-centered. He responds positively to trust and respect for privacy; caution caregivers to maintain a balance between taking an interest in the adolescent's activities and prying into his affairs.

Because peer-group acceptance is important to the adolescent, he will try to conform in dress, hairstyle, mannerisms, habits, and musical tastes. For some adolescents, the need for acceptance may lead to the development of some undesirable behaviors. If the child is not selective of his friends and has a weak self-concept, he may become involved in using tobacco, alcohol, or drugs or engage in sexual relationships to gain acceptance. A positive role identity can help him resist such activities.

Hospitalization threatens the adolescent's independence. If placed on a regular pediatric unit instead of an adolescent unit, he may resent being on a "children's floor"; therefore, he should be allowed extra privileges over the younger children on the unit.

Adolescents fear losing control in the presence of peers. In the hospital, painful procedures should be performed in a private area, away from peers if possible.

Cognition. Piaget's theory contends that, during adolescence, concrete thinking gives way to formal operations; the adolescent becomes fully capable of logical thought and reasoning. He questions adult moral values—no longer accepting them blindly—and will note any inconsistencies in such values; at this time, he may want to discuss any internal conflicts openly with an adult. He also may become actively involved in causes and idealistic movements.

Language. The adolescent's language skills are at an adult level; however, his speech may be colored with slang or other jargon commonly used among his peers. In the hospital setting, avoid speaking to the child using peer-group expressions.

Also at this age, the adolescent has an adult concept of death. He can communicate his feelings about death maturely.

Nursing considerations

Medication. Adolescents usually cooperate with medication administration in an adult manner. Because the deltoid muscles are developed at this age, they may be used for I.M. injections.

Nutrition. During adolescence, boys usually experience at least 1 year of extreme body growth; in girls, this usually occurs during the prepubertal period. Typically, adolescent boys eat constantly during this period.

Caloric requirements are only broad recommendations; individual needs are usually based on activity level (see *Caloric requirements for the pediatric patient*). Athletic adolescents require extra calories from foods high in nutritional value, not "empty" calories from junk food. Milk is usually the liquid of choice at this age because of the adolescent's need for extra calcium.

CALORIC REQUIREMENTS FOR THE PEDIATRIC PATIENT

The average distribution of calories needed for a well-balanced diet are as follows:
• 50% carbohydrates
• 35% fat
• 15% protein.

Below is a breakdown of the normal daily requirements for children of all ages. Keep in mind that, during adolescence, caloric needs will vary, depending on the child's participation in sports and other activities.

Classification	Age	Daily requirements
Neonatal	0 to 1 month	115 to 120 calories/kg
Infant	1 month to 1 year	100 to 110 calories/kg
Toddler	1 to 3	100 to 105 calories/kg
Preschool age	3 to 6	90 to 95 calories/kg
Middle childhood	6 to 11	85 to 90 calories/kg
Prepubertal	11 to 13	Boys: 55 to 65 calories/kg Girls: 45 to 55 calories/kg
Adolescent	13 to 18	Boys: 40 to 50 calories/kg Girls: 35 to 40 calories/kg

In the hospital, allow adolescents their favorite foods from home or peers, if permitted. Some foods often considered junk foods, such as pizza, tacos, and hamburgers, are actually nutritious. Keep high-quality snacks on hand in the unit refrigerator.

During adolescence, some children begin to develop poor eating habits that can lead to serious eating disorders, such as anorexia nervosa and bulimia. Obesity, caused by overeating, underactivity, or both, also may begin to develop at this time. Encourage children with such problems to work out a diet plan and refer them for counseling, if needed.

Safety considerations. Most adolescent deaths result from accidents. At this age, children have a tendency to be impulsive and aggressive. Trying to impress their peers, they may feel indestructible and sometimes show off, inadvertently causing accidents.

Some so-called accidents may be deliberate. Adolescence is a high-risk age for suicide; alert caregivers to the signs of depression and suicidal tendencies and encourage them to promote positive behaviors.

Other common accidents include those associated with sports, swimming, driving, improper use of guns, and drug overdose. At this time, booster immunizations are due and should be encouraged, especially to prevent tetanus.

Participation of the primary caregiver. During the child's adolescent stage, caregivers should not expect to room-in during hospitalization. Frequent visits, however, are usually appreciated, even though the child may be reluctant to admit so. Provide privacy for visits.

Although some caregivers may enjoy the child's return to a state of dependency during the illness or hospitalization, they should be encouraged to help the child maintain a sense of independence. Help the caregiver to let go by encouraging the pursuit of outside interests. Also suggest that the caregiver act as the child's liaison with school, helping with homework and other assignments.

Keep in mind that caregivers face certain financial responsibilities associated with the child's hospitalization and expect regular progress reports on the child's condition. Also, they need to be included in discharge planning. During such planning, stress the importance of keeping a balance between the child's dependency on the caregiver and his need for maintaining self-care.

☐ Admission assessment

Regardless of the child's age, when taking the initial pediatric assessment, keep in mind the following guidelines:
• Provide a quiet, private setting in which to take the patient history and perform the physical assessment. Be sure to move slowly and speak softly.
• When introducing yourself to the child and his caregivers, explain that the information you obtain from the patient history and physical assessment will help tailor nursing care to the child's individual needs. (They may question the necessity of repeating certain information and undergoing procedures already performed during the medical assessment.)
• Establish eye contact, especially when speaking with the child.
• Identify which caregiver is the child's primary caregiver. (Do not automatically assume this is the child's mother.)
• Communicate with the child as well as with the caregivers. This will help you to establish a rapport with the child and obtain helpful information if the child is old enough to talk.
• Avoid using medical terminology. Be informal, but don't digress from the subject.
• Try to appear unhurried and be a good listener. Give the caregivers a chance to express their concerns. *Remember:* In pediatric nursing, the "patient" is the family.
• Use open-ended questions when taking the history; document information in the same words the child or caregivers use, when appropriate.
• Remain open-minded, accepting, and nonjudgmental throughout the history-taking and physical assessment process.

Patient history

The initial patient history is usually comprehensive. Most hospitals provide an assessment form on which to document essential

IMMUNIZATION SEQUENCE

Age	Vaccination
2 months	Diptheria-tetanus-pertussis (DTP) (first dose), polio (first dose)
4 months	DTP (second dose), polio (second dose)
6 months	DTP (third dose)
15 months	Measles, mumps, rubella
18 months	DTP (fourth dose), polio (third dose)
24 months	*Hemophilus influenzae* type B, pneumococcus*
4 to 5 years	DTP (fifth dose), polio (fourth dose)

*Recommended but not required.

information. The major areas covered in the history are listed below.

Identifying information. This information typically includes the child's name, date of birth, address, religion, sex, the name the child responds to, the name and relationship of those providing the information, and the date on which the interview took place.

Chief complaint. This information explains, in the child's or caregiver's words, the reason for the hospitalization.

History of present illness. This information explores the chief complaint in terms of chronology, severity, relief measures, aggravating or precipitating factors, associated symptoms, region, radiation, frequency of occurrence, and any other pertinent information.

Past medical history. The child's past medical history, like an adult's history, should include any previous medical problems. It also should include information about the child's prenatal status, birth, postnatal factors, immunizations, and childhood illnesses (see *Immunization sequence,* and *Common communicable diseases,* pages 32 to 34).

Medications and allergies. Included is such information as the drug name, dosage, time schedule, and patient response to all medications. Be sure to ask about over-the-counter medications; many caregivers forget to mention these because they don't think of them as medications.

Habits and daily activities. Ask the caregivers the following questions, depending on the child's age and developmental level:
Diet and elimination
• How is the child's appetite?
• Is he on a formula? If so, what type?
• When are his usual mealtimes?

(continued on page 35)

COMMON COMMUNICABLE DISEASES

Below is a list of some common communicable diseases and infections of childhood along with their usual signs and symptoms and nursing considerations.

	Signs and symptoms	Nursing considerations
Parotitis (mumps)	Prodromal symptoms that last for 24 hours, including myalgia, anorexia, malaise, headache, and a low-grade fever; followed by an earache, parotid gland tenderness and swelling, a temperature of 101° to 104° F. (38.3° to 40° C.), and pain when chewing or drinking. Swelling of one or more of the salivary glands also may occur.	• Incubation usually is 18 days but may range from 12 to 26 days. • Child is contagious until all swelling disappears; respiratory isolation is recommended until all symptoms subside. • Restrict the child to bed rest until fever subsides. • Administer analgesics and apply compresses to the neck to relieve pain. • Administer antipyretics and give tepid sponge baths for fever. • Encourage the child to drink plenty of fluids to prevent dehydration. • During the acute phase, observe the child closely for central nervous system involvement (such as altered level of consciousness and nuchal rigidity). • Stress to caregivers the importance of immunization at age 15 months and for susceptible children (especially boys) who are approaching or are past puberty. (*Note:* Immunization within 24 hours after exposure may prevent or attenuate the actual disease. Immunity lasts at least 12 years.)
Pertussis (whooping cough)	• After an incubation period of 7 to 10 days, *Bordetella pertussis* enters the tracheobronchial mucosa, where it produces tenacious mucus. This is followed by a classic course of whooping cough, which occurs in three stages, each lasting about 2 weeks. • In the *catarrhal* stage, the child characteristically has an irritating and hacking nocturnal cough, anorexia, sneezing, listlessness, infected conjunctiva, and (occasionally) a low-grade fever. This stage is highly communicable. • After about 1 to 2 weeks, the *paroxysmal* stage produces spasmodic and recurrent coughing that may expel tenacious mucus. Each cough ends in a characteristically loud, crowing inspiratory whoop; choking on mucus causes vomiting. (Newborns and young infants may not develop the typical whoop.) • During the *convalescent* stage, paroxysmal coughing and vomiting gradually subside. However, for months afterward, even a mild upper respiratory infection may trigger coughing.	• Institute aggressive supportive care and respiratory isolation throughout the illness. • Administer fluid and electrolyte replacement, as ordered. Monitor acid-base, fluid, and electrolyte levels. • Administer codeine, mild sedatives, antibiotics, and oxygen, as ordered. • Carefully suction secretions and monitor oxygen therapy. (*Note:* Suctioning removes oxygen as well as secretions.) • Create a quiet environment to decrease coughing stimulation. • Provide small, frequent meals. • Treat constipation or nausea caused by codeine. • To decrease exposure to organisms, change soiled linens, empty the suction bottle, and change the trash bag at least once per shift.

COMMON COMMUNICABLE DISEASES (continued)

	Signs and symptoms	Nursing considerations
Roseola infantum	• After a 10- to 15-day incubation period, the infant develops an abruptly rising fever and, sometimes, seizures. Temperature peaks at 103° to 105° F. (39.4° to 40.6° C.) for 3 to 5 days, then suddenly drops. • During the early febrile period, the infant may be anorexic, irritable, and listless, but does not seem particularly ill. • Simultaneously with the sudden drop in temperature, a maculopapular, nonpruritic rash develops profusely on the trunk, arms, and neck and mildly on the face and legs. The rash fades within 24 hours.	• Administer antipyretics and give tepid sponge baths to lower fever. • If necessary, administer anticonvulsants, as ordered, to relieve seizures. (Seizures usually cease after fever subsides.) • Make sure the infant receives adequate fluid intake.
Rubella (German measles)	• In young children, after an incubation period of 16 to 18 days, an exanthematous maculopapular rash erupts suddenly. • In adolescents, prodromal symptoms—headache, malaise, anorexia, low-grade fever (99° to 101° F. [37.2° to 38.3° C.], coryza, lymphadenopathy, and (sometimes) conjunctivitis—appear before the rash. • Rash usually begins on the face, spreads rapidly, and covers the trunk and extremities within hours. Small, red, petechial macules on the soft palate may precede or accompany the rash. By the end of the 2nd day, the rash on the face begins to fade; however, the rash on the trunk may be confluent and possibly mistaken for scarlet fever. The rash usually disappears on the 3rd day, but may persist for 4 to 5 days. • Suboccipital, postauricular, and postcervical lymph node enlargement usually occurs.	• Make the child as comfortable as possible. Give him books to read or games to play to keep him occupied. • Institute respiratory isolation during the contagious phase (about 10 days before to 5 days after rash appears). • Administer antipyretics to reduce fever. • Do not expose the child to pregnant women while he is contagious. (Transplacental transmission, especially in the first trimester, can cause serious birth defects.)
Rubeola (measles)	• Prodromal symptoms (beginning about 11 days after exposure to the disease) include fever, photophobia, malaise, anorexia, conjunctivitis, coryza, hoarseness, and hacking cough. • After the prodromal phase, Koplik's spots (tiny bluish-gray specks surrounded by a red halo) appear on the oral mucosa opposite the molars. • About 5 days after the appearance of Koplik's spots, temperature rises sharply, spots slough off, and a slightly pruritic rash appears. This characteris-	• Incubation period usually is 10 to 14 days. • The child is contagious from 4 days before until 5 days after rash appears. • Make sure the child receives plenty of rest and increased fluids. • Administer antipyretics and tepid sponge baths to reduce fever. • Observe for signs and symptoms of complications, including encephalitis, otitis media, and pneumonia. • Administer gamma globulin, if ordered, to lighten the attack. (This also

(continued)

COMMON COMMUNICABLE DISEASES (continued)

	Signs and symptoms	Nursing considerations
Rubeola (continued)	tic rash starts as faint macules behind the ears and on the neck and cheeks. These macules become papular and erythematous, rapidly spreading over the entire face, neck, eyelids, arms, chest, back, abdomen, and thighs. When the rash reaches the feet (usually 2 to 3 days later), it begins to fade in the same sequence as it appeared, leaving a brownish discoloration that disappears within 7 to 10 days. • About 2 to 3 days after the rash appears, the child develops fever of 103° to 105° F. (39.4° to 40.6° C.), severe cough, puffy red eyes, and rhinorrhea. • About 5 days after the rash appears, other symptoms disappear and communicability ends.	may be given prophylactically to prevent the disease.) Immunity to the disease develops after one attack.
Streptococcal pharyngitis (strep throat)	• After a 1- to 5-day incubation period, symptoms include temperature of 101° to 104° F. (38.3° to 40° C.), sore throat with severe pain on swallowing, beefy red pharynx, tonsillar exudate, edematous tonsils and uvula, swollen glands along the jaw line, generalized malaise and weakness, anorexia, and occasional abdominal discomfort. • Up to 40% of small children have symptoms too mild for diagnosis. • Fever subsides in 3 to 5 days; nearly all symptoms subside within 1 week.	• Administer penicillin or erythromycin, as ordered. • Institute bed rest and isolation from other children for 24 hours after antibiotic therapy begins. • Make sure the child receives the complete course of treatment, even if symptoms subside. • Scarlet fever (marked by a fine rash on the body) may follow streptococcal pharyngitis.
Varicella (chicken pox)	Prodromal symptoms, including mild fever, malaise, and anorexia; followed in 24 to 36 hours by crops of small, erythematous macules on the trunk or scalp that progress to papules and then clear vesicles on an erythematous base. The vesicles become cloudy and break easily; then scabs form. Occasionally, shallow ulcers form on the mucous membranes of the mouth, conjunctivae, and genitalia.	• The incubation period for chicken pox is 2 to 3 weeks, usually 13 to 17 days. • Child is contagious for 6 days after rash appears. (Scabs are not infectious.) • Administer local or systemic antipruritics, as ordered. • Trim fingernails to prevent scratching. Apply a paste of baking soda and water (or alcohol) to ease itching. • Observe for signs of complications, including severe skin pain and burning. • Do not admit a child exposed to the disease to a unit containing children who receive immunosuppressants or who have leukemia or immunodeficiency disorders. • Administer varicella-zoster immunoglobulin, as ordered, to susceptible children who have been exposed to the disease to help lessen its severity. • Immunity develops after one attack.

• Does he eat with family members?
• Does someone usually help him eat?
• Does he use utensils?
• Does he have any difficulty eating? If so, what sort?
• What are his favorite foods and beverages?
• Does he snack? What does he usually have for snacks?
• Does he take vitamins?
• Is he toilet trained? At what age did he learn?
• What are his usual bowel habits?
• Does he wet the bed?

Exercise and sleep
• Does his daily schedule include play?
• Does he participate in sports?
• Does he perform any special exercises regularly?
• What is his normal amount of sleep? What time does he get up and go to bed?
• Does he take naps?
• Does he have a routine before going to sleep (such as drinking a bottle, playing, or being read to)?
• Does he sleep with siblings or alone?
• What is his favorite sleeping position?
• Does he have any sleeping problems? Any nightmares?
• Is he tired during the day?

Recreation
• How much time does he get for recreation each day?
• Does he have a group of friends with whom he plays?
• What are his favorite play activities?

Family history. Try to trace at least two generations of medical disorders.

Developmental history. Review with the caregiver the child's major developmental milestones (such as rolling over, standing, and walking); also note the age at which they were accomplished.

Systems review. Ask the caregivers if the child has ever complained about (or if the caregivers have been aware of any of the following problems):
• Eyes: vision difficulties, problems with tearing, crossed eyes
• Ears: hearing difficulties, earaches
• Nose: nosebleeds, sinus infections
• Throat: sore throats (especially streptococcal), colds (more than four per year)
• Cardiovascular: bluish skin color, fatigue
• Respiratory: breathing difficulties, shortness of breath, frequent exhaustion
• GI: changes in bowel habits, diarrhea, constipation, bleeding, pain, vomiting
• Renal: frequent urination, pain, bleeding on urination, problems with urine flow (with boys)

• Reproductive: premature onset of menstruation
• Neurologic: headaches, seizures (febrile or nonfebrile), tremors, twitches, dizziness, loss of consciousness
• Musculoskeletal: painful joints, redness around joints, swelling, sprains, broken bones, coordination difficulties.

Physical assessment

Depending on the child's age and temperament, performing a physical assessment may be difficult. Keeping the child's developmental characteristics in mind will help; however, flexibility in approach will be your key to success. Each child is an individual and won't always behave according to his age or developmental group, so remember to take your cues from the child himself.

When performing the physical assessment, keep in mind the following points:
• To avoid seeming large and overwhelming to the child, try to position yourself so that you are at eye level with him, at least initially. You may need to sit in a chair or on a stool to do this.
• Do not undress the child yourself. Depending on his age, allow him to undress himself or have his caregiver do it for him; this causes less stress to the child. Also, minimize the amount of time the child is undressed, and undress only the body area to be examined at one time.
• Before performing auscultation, palpation, and percussion, always warm your hands and any needed equipment, including the diaphragm of the stethoscope.
• Perform the least invasive steps first.
• Be alert to signs of abuse, such as bruises, scars, and burns, regardless of the child's age or developmental level. This is considered a major area of responsibility in pediatric nursing.
• Throughout the assessment process, make generalized obervations about the child's reactions to and relationships with his caregivers. Such abnormal behaviors as overt hostility or submissiveness, withdrawal, attention-seeking activities, or disturbed speech patterns could indicate problems of abuse or neglect.

The physical assessment usually begins with measurement of the child's vital signs and his height, weight, and head and chest circumferences (head circumference is measured in children up to age 2; chest circumference is measured in infants). Height, weight, and head circumference should be plotted on an age-appropriate growth grid to assess the child's progress or risk status in comparison with other children (see the "Physical Growth Charts" in the Appendices).

The next step in the assessment process involves examining the child using either a cephalocaudal (head-to-toe) or body systems approach. Keep in mind that your approach and expected findings will depend to a great extent on the child's developmental level. Assessment variations based on the developmental framework discussed earlier in this section are provided below.

Neonatal period (birth to age 1 month)

General appearance. Note skin color and turgor. Observe for alertness and activity level.

Measurements. When taking the child's vital signs, begin by counting respirations, the least invasive measurement. Before taking the apical pulse, remember to warm your hands and the stethoscope. Keep in mind that newborns have a rapid heart rate that may be difficult to count. Take your time to make sure the count is accurate, and remember to listen for the rhythm.

Be aware of your institution's policy regarding the recommended route for temperature measurement. As a general rule, a rectal temperature is contraindicated if the child has diarrhea. Always use great caution when taking a newborn's rectal temperature because of the potential for damaging the tiny bowel.

To take a rectal temperature, insert the tip of the thermometer just inside the internal anal sphincter and hold the thermometer in place. To take an axillary temperature, place the thermometer vertically along the newborn's trunk with the tip well into the axilla (see *Vital sign measurements,* page 23).

Next, measure the newborn's height, weight, and head and chest circumferences. Plot these measurements on a growth grid and compare these findings with the norms (see "Physical Growth Charts" in the Appendices).

Head and face. Check the entire head region for symmetry. Then, palpate the fontanelles, noting size, shape, bulges, and depressions. To help estimate fontanelle size, you should know the width of your own index and middle finger in centimeters.

Check for uncoordinated eye movements, which may stem from immaturity; reassure the caregivers that this is not unusual with newborns. Note any crusty material on the eyelids and remove it with sterile water. Inspect the mouth and gums for signs of oral candidiasis (thrush), which presents as white patches resembling milk curds; these patches, unlike milk curds, are not easily dislodged when swabbed.

Chest. Keep in mind that newborns are nose breathers. Retractions of the chest indicate respiratory distress; during your assessment, be sure to note the area of retraction (such as the substernal, suprasternal, or intercostal area).

Abnormal chest sounds may indicate nasal congestion (transmitted sounds). Clean the newborn's nose with a bulb syringe, offer him some water (if allowed), then listen again.

Abdomen. Carefully observe and smell the umbilical cord for inflammation, purulent drainage, and foul odor. Umbilical hernias are not unusual.

Genitalia. With boys, check for circumcision healing. Note the location of the urinary meatus; however, do not forcibly retract the foreskin if the newborn is uncircumcised. Hydrocele, not uncommon, can be differentiated from variocele or hernia by transillumination. Also remember to palpate the testes with one hand by trapping each testicle in the scrotal sac with the other hand (see "Genitourinary and reproductive systems" in Section 2 for a further explanation).

With girls, vaginal bleeding or discharge is not unusual; reassure caregivers that this is a normal response to maternal hormones and will subside.

Neurologic and musculoskeletal systems. Observe the newborn for muscle tone; muscles should not be flaccid or spastic. Also check for presence of neonatal reflexes, such as the Moro, sucking, rooting, grasp, tonic neck, and crawling reflexes.

Infant period (age 1 month to 1 year)

Approach. Usually, infants under age 6 months present little difficulty during an assessment; however, after age 6 months, infants begin developing characteristics that could pose certain difficulties. For example, infants typically have a short attention span. They are easily startled and highly sensitive to environmental stimuli. They also develop stranger anxiety.

Perform the assessment with the child positioned securely on the caregiver's lap. Being as efficient as possible, move slowly and smoothly to avoid triggering an outburst.

Allow the caregivers to do the undressing. Usually, the infant will be cooperative and may even enjoy being undressed. However, if the infant is uncooperative during the examination, reassure the caregivers that this is normal for the child's developmental level.

General information. Keep in mind the following information during the examination:
• Check the infant's alertness and responsiveness by making expressive faces at him and speaking to him, then observing for his reactions.
• Because obtaining a blood pressure reading may be difficult, try using the Doppler or flush method instead of the conventional method (see *Taking a child's blood pressure,* page 21).
• "Baby fat" usually develops at an increasing rate during the first 9 months, then begins to decrease.

Head. The fontanelles should be flat, with no bulges or depressions. The anterior fontanelle should be diamond-shaped and open; the posterior fontanelle should close within 4 to 8 weeks after birth. Assess for any bulges with the infant upright and quiet.

Skull sutures may be palpated as ridges until the infant is about age 8 months. Auscultation of bruits is not uncommon at this age. Measure head circumference and plot the measurement on a graph. Transillumination may be used if the skull is large.

Cradle cap (seborrheic dermatitis), a common condition, is preventable with daily head washing. Provide caregivers with treatment instructions, if needed, and reassure them that washing the scalp will not damage the infant's "soft spots."

Head control usually begins when the infant is about age 3 months; the head should be stable by age 5 months.

Eyes. Check the infant's red reflex to rule out cataracts or corneal opacity. Transient strabismus is normal during infancy. Tearing is uncommon before age 3 months because of immaturity of the tear apparatus. Note the child's permanent eye color (usually achieved by age 1 year).

Ears. An infant age 6 months or older usually turns to hear his caregiver's voice and progresses from cooing to babbling and other speech sounds. Failure to turn to hear the caregiver's voice or babbling in monotone may indicate hearing loss.

When examining the infant's ears, pull the pinnae down and back and insert an otoscope speculum ¼″ to ½″ (0.6 to 1.3 cm).

Oral cavity. During your assessment, keep in mind that infants generally resent examination of the oral cavity. Examining this area early in the assessment process may mean losing the infant's cooperation for the remainder of the examination. For this reason, examine the oral cavity last.

The first teeth to erupt are the lower central incisors, usually at about age 5 or 6 months. By age 1 year, he should have six teeth. During the teething period, drooling and irritability are normal. Comfort measures include teething rings, massage, and applying cold compresses to the area.

Neck. Because the infant's neck is extremely short, you'll need to extend it for palpation.

Chest. Usually rounded, the infant's chest should be measured for the first 9 months. Chest circumference measurements, usually taken at the nipple line during midrespiration, may reveal anomalies, birth injuries, or cardiac enlargement.

The infant may have hypertrophy of the breast for the first 3 months. Crying may be used to assess thrills in the child's chest.

Heart. During auscultation, expect to hear a split S_2 heart sound and normal sinus arrhythmia.

Abdomen. Respirations are abdominal in infancy. Be sure to report any intercostal respiratory movement, which indicates respiratory distress.

Umbilical hernia, common in infants, usually closes spontaneously by age 2 in white children, later in black children. Reassure caregivers that closure will occur. The liver is normally palpable 1 to 2 cm below the right costal margin.

Musculoskeletal system. Keep in mind that an infant cannot follow instructions to demonstrate range of motion. Perform passive range of motion to songs or rhymes to relax the child.

Infants typically appear flat-footed, usually because of normal fat pad distribution. Because hip dysplasia may not be evident during the neonatal period, assessment for this condition should continue during the first year (see "Hip dysplasia" under the "Neuromuscular and musculoskeletal systems" heading in Section 2 for signs and symptoms). Bowleggedness is not unusual until the child is approximately age 18 months.

Neurologic system. Expect the achievement of many developmental milestones during the infant's first year, indicating an intact nervous system. Persistence of infant reflexes after age 4 months indicates abnormality. Protective reflexes, such as the parachute and tripod, should emerge at about age 6 months.

Genitourinary system. The foreskin of an uncircumcised infant normally is tight until about age 3 to 4 months. Never forcibly retract the foreskin. Report any tightness that persists beyond age 4 months.

Toddler period (age 1 to 3)

Approach. Be prepared for wide variations in cooperation among toddlers. Some actually enjoy the examination process and cooperate fully, whereas others offer little or no cooperation. Remember that toddlers have the strength and mobility to resist by kicking, biting, or running away.

Take advantage of the child's growing curiosity about his surroundings. Attract his attention with dolls, puppets, teddy bears, and other toys. Use them to acquaint him with the equipment you will be using. Whatever distraction method you use, keep in mind that the toddler's attention span is short. Use your judgment about how long to play with him.

During the examination, allow the toddler to sit on his caregiver's lap or to stand at the caregiver's side. If the procedure requires a reclining position, have the child lie across the caregiver's lap. If the child is quiet, auscultate his chest and abdomen first, leaving for last any procedures that are likely to upset him.

General information. By age 3, the child's head will be 75% that of adult size (see "Physical Growth Charts" in the Appendices). Respirations during this age are abdominal (see *Taking a child's blood pressure,* page 21, and *Vital sign measurements,* page 23.)

Eyes. By age 1, the child's eye muscles should function with good coordination. Persistent strabismus requires medical attention to prevent amblyopia, which, if uncorrected by age 3 to 4, may result in vision loss (see *Visual acuity: What's normal?,* page 7).

Ears. To examine the toddler's ears, pull the pinnae down and back to straighten the external auditory canals. Suspect hearing impairment if the child:
• fails to speak clearly by age 2
• habitually yells or shrieks when playing or communicating
• responds to facial expressions rather than words
• appears shy or withdrawn or prefers playing by himself
• seems inattentive, dreamy, or stubborn
• often looks confused or puzzled
• lacks interest in hearing stories and nursery rhymes or in playing vocal games, such as riddles.

Oral cavity. By age 18 to 24 months, a child usually has 16 deciduous teeth. By 30 months, primary dentition is complete with 20 deciduous teeth. To remember the number of teeth to expect in a child under age 2, subtract 6 from the child's age in months.

Instruct caregivers in the importance of a proper diet and oral hygiene for children of this age-group. If the child is not weaned by age 1, he should be given only water in his bottle before bedtime or naptime to prevent "bottle mouth caries." Daily care should include brushing teeth.

Enlarged tonsils are not unusual in children of this age-group.

Nose. When examining the child's nose, observe for nasal flaring, an indication of respiratory distress. Also look for nasal polyps or other deformities. (Nasal polyps often are present in children who live with cigarette smokers. Discuss this with the caregivers.)

Chest. Expect the lateral diameter to surpass the anteroposterior diameter as the overall chest circumference increases. Remember to observe for deformities and retractions (intercostal, suprasternal, and substernal).

Hyperresonance is normal at this age. Breath sounds over lung fields are bronchovesicular. By age 2, the apex of the heart should be at the fifth left intercostal space.

Abdomen. The toddler usually is potbellied. The child's own fingers may be used to palpate the abdominal area if he is ticklish or frightened. The liver may be palpable up to three fingerbreadths below the costal margin.

Musculoskeletal system. During this stage, the toddler's legs are elongating. At age 1, the legs may appear bowed because of the child's shortness and the weight of a disproportionately large trunk; by age 3, this bowed look will disappear.

Neurologic system. Expect a positive Babinski reflex until the child begins walking.

Preschool period (age 3 to 6)

Approach. Preschoolers are usually cooperative and eager to please. At a stage when they are developing initiative, they sometimes enjoy being the center of attention and may feel that being examined on a table is like being "on stage." Always allow the preschooler to choose where he wants to sit for the examination, such as on the bed, chair, or table or on the caregiver's lap.

Because prechoolers enjoy teasing and play, incorporate playfulness into your approach. For example, when examining the child's ears, you might say, "Let's look for frogs in your ears."

Also keep in mind that, at this stage, the child understands simple explanations and commands. Tell (don't ask) him what you want him to do to help. For example, you might say, "Now take off your shirt so I can listen to your heart." Then, praise and flatter him for doing as you asked.

General information. The preschooler's proportion of body fat generally decreases at this age. By age 5 to 6, the child's head has achieved 90% of adult size. Preschoolers are advanced to the second level (age 2 to 18) of the growth grid (see "Physical Growth Charts" in the Appendices).

Note the following information:
• Blood pressure measurements are essential over age 3.
• Oral temperature measurement usually is not possible before age 5, except with an electronic thermometer.
• Immunizations should be given routinely; remind parents about immunization requirements for school enrollment.

Head. Because of their tendency for close interactive play, preschoolers are prone to transmission of head lice and scalp infections. Be on the alert for signs of nits, scratching, or excoriation.

Eyes. The preschooler is at greatest risk of developing amblyopia at age 4. Careful screening and intervention may avert permanent vision loss (see *Visual acuity: What's normal?,* page 7).

Ears. Speech development depends on early detection of hearing loss. Testing with tuning forks, audiometry, and tympanometry is useful and children seem to enjoy it. Creative approaches to hearing assessment may include having the child identify the sounds of toys.

Although some cerumen is normal, dark impacted cerumen may indicate improper cleaning techniques. Discourage caregivers from inserting cotton-tipped applicators into the child's ears.

Oral cavity. Observe the child for bite defects and dental caries. Enlarged tonsils are not abnormal at this age.

Encourage caregivers to promote good oral hygiene. Visits to the dentist should begin during the preschool years.

Nose. Nasal polyps or signs of allergy may be caused by exposure to smoking in the home. Provide teaching as needed.

Chest. The transverse-anteroposterior diameter is approaching the adult index at this age; abnormal chest development may indicate a chronic respiratory disorder.

S_3 heart sounds may occur in preschoolers; report these, if heard, for further evaluation. An irregular pulse also may occur. Blood pressure increases slightly at this stage (see *Taking a child's blood pressure,* page 21, for normal ranges).

Abdomen. The potbellied appearance characteristic of the toddler years gradually diminishes during the preschool years. By age 5, the torso is usually slim. The liver may be palpable.

If the child complains of abdominal pain, ask him to locate the site by pointing to it with one finger. Keep in mind that the closer he points to the umbilicus, the more likely the pain is not organic in origin. Find out when the pain occurs in relation to activities and time of day. This is a critical part of the child's history of abdominal pain.

Rectal area. Perform a digital examination only if indicated by the child's history. Report any discharge, irritation, and dilatation; these may indicate possible abuse.

Neuromuscular and musculoskeletal systems. During the preschool years, expect a slower rate of physical growth (most of the child's height gain will be in the legs) with development of increased strength, skill, and coordination (gross and fine motor); also expect the child to have established handedness. The physical examination should include assessment for spinal deformities, such as scoliosis, kyphosis, and lordosis.

Provide a hospitalized child with puzzles and coloring and drawing activities; these provide much enjoyment, require little energy, and encourage evolving neuromuscular skills.

Middle childhood (age 6 to 11)

Approach. Children in this age group are often curious, interested, and capable of following directions. They want to please and thrive on flattery. When examining such a child, give simple, precise instructions using age-appropriate vocabulary. Then praise the child for his cooperation.

Older children in this age-group are developing a sense of modesty; remember this during your examination.

General information. Keep in mind the following information:
• Take the child's temperature by either the oral or axillary route; rectal temperatures, frequently resisted by children of this age-group, usually are unnecessary.
• Conversation about school and friends provides a good indication of the child's overall adjustment. Remember, these are often the healthiest years of life.

Head. By age 6, the child's head is about 90% of adult size.

Eyes. A Snellen chart is used to test the child's eyesight; an E chart may be required for children age 5 to 6. A good internal eye examination also is a useful tool; however, this usually is not considered a nursing responsibility.

By age 10, epicanthal folds have disappeared in non-Oriental children.

Ears. During this age, the pinnae grow in proportion to the child's head.

If the child has a history of frequent attacks of otitis media, hearing tests are extremely important. To test hearing, use the whisper test: Whisper simple questions to the child from a distance of 8' (2.4 m), making sure to use words he knows and not letting him see your lips. Tuning fork tests and audiometric testing (not always available) may also be used; children in this age-group usually enjoy these tests.

Also remember to listen to the child's speech; speech development reflects hearing ability. By age 7, the child should be articulating correctly.

Oral cavity. Children in this age-group sometimes dread oral examinations and noticeably relax once the procedure is over. For this reason, consider performing the oral examination first in the assessment procedure and attempt to examine the child without using a tongue depressor.

During middle childhood, tonsils are normally enlarged. The first permanent molars should appear at about age 6. Gaps from loss of deciduous teeth are also normal; teeth usually are replaced in the same order as deciduous eruptions. Reinforce the need for good dental hygiene.

Chest. By age 7, respirations change to thoracic in girls; boys continue with abdominal breathing. Breast budding, frequently unilateral at first, may begin at age 9 in girls; boys remain flat-chested. Instruction on breast self-examination techniques should begin at this time.

Heart. The child may have an irregular rhythm, which is within normal limits. When the child is asked to hold his breath, the pulse should become regular.

Abdomen. Because the child tends to swallow air, tympany will be louder than in an adult. A lordotic stance makes the child appear potbellied.

Neurologic system. Transient tics are not unusual. If present, note the history of onset, duration, and any other relevant information; however, obtain this information from the caregivers out of the child's hearing. Avoid drawing attention to the tic.

Prepubertal period (age 11 to 13)

Approach. Ask the prepubertal child if he prefers having his parents in the room during the examination. Provide him with a gown to wear during the examination, and allow him to undress privately.

During the assessment, explain what you are doing and why. Encourage him to ask questions, and answer them honestly. Keep in mind that he may be self-conscious and easily embarrassed. Examine the child's genitalia last, when he is more at ease with you. If appropriate, reassure him that everything appears normal.

General information. A prepubertal child may have a slightly chubby appearance, a normal finding for this transitional stage.

Teeth. During this age, the child will have lost the last of his deciduous teeth; 12-year molars begin to erupt. Orthodontia, if needed, is usually started at this time.

Sexual maturity. Prepubertal children usually fall within Tanner's Stage I or II of sexual maturity (refer to a primary pediatrics textbook for further information).

With boys, expect wide variations in speed of maturation. Typical findings during the examination include:
• enlarged testes and a longer penis
• long, fine pubic hair
• red and corrugated scrotal skin
• no axillary or facial hair.

The child and caregivers need to be informed about the normalcy of individual variations concerning the onset and speed of maturation. Teach the child to do monthly testicular examinations. (Suggest that he use his birthdate each month as a reminder to do the examination).

With girls, typical examination findings include:
• elevation of the breasts
• long, fine, straight pubic hair
• thickened labia
• no axillary hair
• menarche (usually occurs between the time the child develops pubic hair and axillary hair; average age in the United States is 12½).

Provide adequate information about sexual development and dispel any myths or misconceptions the child may have. Teach breast self-examination and prepare her for the possibility of irregular menstrual cycles during the first 2 years after menarche.

Musculoskeletal system. Prepubertal children often appear clumsy; this is because the skeletal system is growing rapidly while the muscles lag behind. (Avoid calling attention to the child's clumsiness.) The extremities usually grow faster than the trunk and head. Poor posture is common, especially with girls, who tend to be taller than boys at this age.

Adolescent period (age 13 to 18)

Approach. Before examining the adolescent, remember to ask whether he wants his caregivers present; he probably will not want them in the room. Provide a gown and allow him to change in private.

As you proceed with the examination, elicit questions and discuss the assessment procedure with him. Keep in mind that he may deny the existence of any health problems and resent being hospitalized, especially if it was done against his will. If this is the case, avoid being drawn into his anger; rather, be warm and friendly, but don't try speaking to him on an adolescent level.

Once you have established a rapport with the adolescent, question him regarding drug use, sexual activity and preferences, and the use of birth control measures (be sure to discuss this out of the caregivers' hearing).

After the examination, review the health problems and care plan with the adolescent. Then decide with him which information to share with his caregivers. Do not violate his trust. If you feel it is necessary to share certain information with the caregivers, even against the child's wishes, be sure to tell him so.

General information. As part of the overall assessment, be sure to note the adolescent's grooming, hygiene, posture, coordination, self-assurance, communication skills, interest in body image and health, and use of eye contact. Because adolescents typically are hygiene-conscious, poor hygienic practices may indicate depression. However, don't mistake trendy attire or an unkempt look for poor hygiene; this is characteristic of adolescence.

Hair and skin. The adolescent may have oily hair and dandruff. He may also have acne on the face, back, and chest. Because appearances are important at this age, be sure to provide teaching on hair and skin care.

Vision. Acuity should be at the normal adult level at this age. Hereditary myopia, frequently associated with a growth spurt, may occur at this time.

Lymph nodes. Palpable lymph nodes, which are more significant in an adolescent than a younger child, usually indicate an active infection or other abnormality.

Teeth. Be sure to check for caries and evidence of good dental hygiene. Also look for malocclusion. Adolescence is the age at which wisdom teeth may be diagnosed as impacted; surgery may be necessary.

Musculoskeletal system. Check for signs of scoliosis.

Breasts and genitalia. In adolescent boys, gynecomastia may occur; be sure to offer reassurance that this condition is not uncommon and usually disappears without treatment as the child matures. In girls, the breasts will show normal enlargement. Remember to teach testicular or breast self-examination during the assessment process.

2 | Diseases and Disorders

Because the nurse often detects signs and symptoms of diseases and disorders during assessment of specific body systems, this section is organized according to body systems. Each body system category includes information on assessment data, including the patient history and physical examination, as well as a discussion of related diseases and disorders you likely will encounter.

☐ Neuromuscular and musculoskeletal systems

Within this category, you likely will encounter a broad range of congenital and acquired conditions. Although only a small sampling of diseases and disorders affecting pediatric patients are discussed here, keep in mind that various disorders of the neuromuscular and musculoskeletal systems have common signs and symptoms. Such signs and symptoms may manifest in subtle ways; congenital problems may not be apparent at birth.

Admission assessment

During the initial assessment, you'll need to collect specific information concerning the child's neuromuscular and musculoskeletal status. Depending on the child's age, you may need to rely on the caretakers as the primary source of information.

Patient history. To establish a sound subjective base for your assessment, ask the following questions, as applicable to the child's developmental level:
• Head: Has the child complained of headaches, dizziness, or vertigo? Does he have a history of trauma or loss of consciousness?
• Neck: Is the child experiencing stiffness or pain?
• Mobility: Does the child have any pain, stiffness, weakness, swelling, or redness around his joints? Does he have limited range of motion, any sign of a limp, or paralysis? Does the child walk? At what age did he begin walking?
• Crepitation: Does a grating sound or sensation occur when a limb is moved?
• Paresthesia or anesthesia: Does the child experience any tingling or loss of sensation?
• Eyes: Does the child have any visual acuity changes or scotoma (gap in the visual field)?
• Speech: How does the child's speech compare with that of his siblings? Does he have a speech impairment? Has his cry changed in pitch?
• Fever: Has the child recently had a fever, rash, or signs of a

minor illness? What medications, including aspirin, were given?
• Involuntary movement: Does the child have any spasms, twitching, tremors, or seizures?
• Bowel and bladder control: Has control been achieved? At what age? Has there been any regression or change?
• Dysphagia: Has the child experienced any choking episodes?
• Activity level: Has the child had any change in his regular activity level? Is he more active or lethargic?
• Ears: Does the child have any deformities or hearing deficit?

Perinatal history. Find out the following information concerning the child's perinatal status:
• During pregnancy: Did the mother experience any trauma or infection or use drugs, alcohol, or tobacco? Was she exposed to X-rays?
• Delivery: How long was the labor? What type of delivery was used? Was there any trauma or use of medications or anesthesia? Is the child's Apgar score known?
• Postnatal: Did the child have any jaundice or breathing problems? Was the suck reflex strong or weak? (Strength of this reflex is a good indication of an infant's strength.) Was the child discharged at the same time as the mother?

Family history. Ask whether there is a family history of seizure disorders, muscular diseases or disorders, cerebral palsy, skeletal deformities, or mental retardation.

Physical assessment
The physical assessment, which should begin the first time you meet the child, includes observing the child's behavior, movement, alertness, and activity level and listening to his speech and cry. Children under age 2 require careful, specialized neurologic evaluation. However, after age 2, the child's neurologic system may be evaluated in a manner similar to that of an adult, except for the creativity and ingenuity required to get his cooperation.

The equipment you'll need to assess the child will vary somewhat from that used to assess an adult. For example, hearing tests will need to be adapted specifically to the child's age. (A sophisticated hearing test that measures auditory evoked brain responses is available for infants, but it requires the use of special equipment and a trained technician. A crude method of testing the infant's hearing may be done by ringing a bell and observing the infant's response.) Also, visual acuity may be tested with age-appropriate charts.

Because delayed development is a common manifestation of neuromuscular and musculoskeletal diseases and disorders, a reliable developmental test kit, such as the Denver Developmental Screening Test (DDST), is a valuable tool for testing children age 6 and younger. The DDST has proved reliable in evaluating children's personal-social, language, and gross and fine motor development.

Reflexes. Although numerous infant reflexes have been identified, the most commonly tested include the following:
• Moro (startle)
• rooting
• sucking
• grasp
• walking (stepping or dancing)
• placing (ladder)
• asymmetrical tonic neck (fencing)
• Babinski (normally positive in infants up to walking age).

Infant reflexes are considered abnormal if they are absent, exaggerated, persistent, or inappropriate for the child's age, or if they reappear after disappearing. Most infant reflexes disappear at approximately age 4 months, when voluntary control develops.

Behavior. The Brazelton Neonatal Behavior Assessment Scale, used to evaluate alertness, motor maturity, irritability, consolableness, and interaction, is especially useful in helping the mother understand her infant's temperament and behavioral characteristics.

Head circumference. Measured up to age 2, head circumference has significant bearing on the child's neurologic status. Directly related to intracranial volume, the head circumference is measured to estimate the rate of brain growth and is used to help diagnose hydrocephalus.

Tremors. Common in newborns, especially during crying episodes, tremors are considered suspicious if they persist, occur at rest, or are localized or of low frequency and high amplitude.

Motor ability and cerebellar function. Children enjoy tests of balance, strength, coordination, and agility; older children especially enjoy resistance games for evaluating muscle strength.

Infant posturing helps to indicate the integrity of the motor system. Up to age 2 months, the child should demonstrate symmetrical semiflexion; after 2 months, extension should be more pronounced. Hip joint stability should be assessed in children under age 1.

To assess the toddler's motor ability, have him walk away from you toward his caregivers (do not suggest that he walk away from his caregivers toward you); be sure to observe his gait, stance, and balance.

Brain tumor

Neoplasms of the brain are less common in children than in adults. However, when they occur, they are usually identified histologically as gliomas, such as the cerebellar astrocytoma type, and are primarily located infratentorially (see *Common intracranial tumors,* page 50).

COMMON INTRACRANIAL TUMORS

Below is a list of some of the most common types of intracranial tumors found in pediatric patients along with defining characteristics and treatment methods.

Tumor type	Defining characteristics	Medical treatment
INFRATENTORIAL		
Brain stem glioma	• Usually an astrocytoma or a glioblastoma • Associated with a high mortality (few children survive beyond age 1) • Cannot be removed surgically because of its location (within vital centers)	• Palliative therapy involving radiation (to shrink tumor and thereby prolong survival)
Cerebellar astrocytoma	• Most common type of brain tumor • Benign (usually cystic) and slow-growing	• Surgical excision (associated with a high rate of cure)
Ependymoma	• Grows at varying speeds • Often occurs in the fourth ventricle, producing cerebrospinal fluid (CSF) obstruction • Can only be removed partially by surgical excision because of its location (close to vital centers)	• Postoperative radiation of the entire craniospinal axis
Medulloblastoma	• Fastest-growing type of brain tumor; highly malignant • Most commonly located in the cerebellum • Difficult to remove surgically	• Radiation and chemotherapy (result in longer survival rates)
SUPRATENTORIAL		
Cerebral tumor	• Usually an astrocytoma or ependymoma • If an astrocytoma: rapid growth rate; invades adjacent structures • If an ependymoma: commonly located in the lateral ventricles • Difficult to remove surgically	• Surgical excision (although success is extremely variable, depending on size, location, and type of tumor) • Radiation and chemotherapy (adjuncts)
Craniopharyngioma	• Most common nongliomatous type of tumor in pediatric patients • Located near the sella turcica • Causes CSF obstruction, disturbed pituitary function, visual problems, and depressed hypothalamic function • May be impossible to remove surgically in its entirety	• Radiation and repeated surgery to reduce tumor size • Hormone replacement (essential)
Optic nerve glioma	• Invades the optic nerve and chiasm • Usually an astrocytoma • Produces variable ocular symptoms, increased intracranial pressure (resulting from obstruction of the foramen of Monro), and atrophy of the optic nerves (resulting from tumor compression)	• Surgical excision (may prolong survival but affects vision)

Clinical manifestations of brain tumors depend on their size and location as well as the developmental stage of the child's skull. Open suture lines may delay the onset of identifiable symptoms.

Assessment

Frequently encountered data for brain tumors include the following:

Subjective

• headache (especially in the early morning)
• nausea
• vomiting (progresses to projectile as intracranial pressure increases)
• visual complaints (such as diplopia)
• vertigo

Objective

• papilledema
• unequal pupils
• behavioral changes (such as irritability, lethargy, or coma)
• enlargement of the head (if sutures are not closed)
• ataxia (if cerebellum is involved)
• seizures
• hyperactive reflexes
• spasticity
• paresis or paralysis
• nystagmus
• unusual posturing of the head (such as tilting to one side)
• changes in vital signs (decrease in pulse and respiratory rates, increase in systolic blood pressure and widened pulse pressure)
• hypothermia or hyperthermia
• localizing signs (related to the cranial nerves or cerebral area affected).

Nursing diagnosis

Altered Comfort: Acute Head Pain related to space-occupying lesion
Desired outcome: The child reports pain relief or demonstrates a return to his usual behavior patterns and play activities.

Interventions

1. Assess the severity, duration, location, and precipitating or aggravating factors associated with the child's pain.
2. Provide a quiet environment and dim lighting.
3. Administer analgesics, as ordered. (Medications that will not mask or alter the child's level of consciousness, such as acetaminophen, usually are given.)
4. Monitor the child's bowel function and take the following measures to avoid constipation and straining at stool:
• Maintain hydration.

• Administer stool softeners, as ordered.
• Avoid using enemas.
5. Explore with the caregivers and child (if appropriate) which positions provide the most comfort, and use them if permitted.

Nursing diagnosis

Sensory-Perceptual Alteration: Visual, Auditory, Kinesthetic, Gustatory, Tactile, or Olfactory Deficit (specify) related to brain tissue injury or pressure on cranial structures secondary to brain tumor
Desired outcome: Sensory deficits are recognized and reversed with treatment and rehabilitation, or the child returns to an optimum level of function.

Interventions

1. Assess and carefully document any deficits in sensory perception. (This information may contribute to the diagnosis and management of the brain tumor.)
2. Provide reality orientation and nonirriting sensory stimulation. For example, tell the child who you are, what day it is, and what his plans for the day are. Also, provide soft music or read quietly to him.
3. Encourage the caregivers to communicate with the child and to provide physical and emotional support regardless of the child's response level.
4. Avoid isolating the child from his peers and the other children on the unit.
5. Provide assistance with prediagnostic and postdiagnostic procedures, as well as with physical and emotional care of the child undergoing treatment (such as surgery, radiation therapy, and chemotherapy).

Nursing diagnosis

Potential for Injury: Trauma related to physical and neurologic factors (such as altered mobility, decreased sensory function, change in level of consciousness, and seizures)
Desired outcome: Risk factors are identified and steps taken to enhance safety.

Interventions

1. Observe the child carefully and perform frequent neurochecks.
2. Keep the crib or bed side rails up.
3. Institute seizure precautions.
4. Maintain the child in the prescribed position; post signs over the crib or bed advising others not to alter this position.
5. Assist the child with hygiene and activities of daily living, encouraging independence whenever possible.
6. Instruct the caregivers in precautionary measures to prevent injury, and enlist their help in monitoring the child's activities.
7. To prevent corneal abrasion, administer liquid tears or apply eye patches or dressings, as needed.

Medical diagnosis

The medical diagnosis for brain tumors is based on:
• the physical examination and patient history
• diagnostic studies. Various combinations of the following studies are used:
   —EEG
   —skull X-rays
   —computed tomography and brain scans
   —arteriography
   —biopsy.

Medical treatment

Surgery is the treatment of choice for most primary brain tumors. If the neoplasm is inoperable or incompletely removed, radiation therapy or antineoplastic chemotherapy is indicated.

Rehabilitation using a multidisciplinary approach is geared toward recovery of lost function.

Cerebral palsy

A chronic, nonprogressive neuromuscular disorder, cerebral palsy is the most common cause of pediatric disability. Effects range from minor to severe dysfunction. Although the specific etiology may be obscure, this disorder essentially results from brain damage caused by infection, trauma, hypoxia, metabolic disease, chemical toxicity, or other factors occurring prenatally, perinatally, or postnatally within the first 5 years of life.

Cerebral palsy is classified according to predominant clinical manifestations:
• spastic—the most common type, marked by hypertonicity, abnormal posture, and muscle weakness
• athetoid—also called dyskinetic; characterized by slow, writhing, involuntary movements that are absent during sleep and aggravated by stress
• ataxic—the least common type, characterized by a lack of coordination caused by an affected cerebellum.

Frequent hospitalizations may occur with this disorder; nurses play an important role in its prevention, detection, and long-term management.

Assessment

Frequently encountered data for cerebral palsy include the following:

Subjective (as reported by caregivers)

• seizures (in 35% of patients)
• strabismus or nystagmus (or both)
• hearing disorders (most common with the athetoid type)
• grimacing, drooling, and writhing movements (most common with the athetoid type) that increase with stress and disappear

with sleep (These signs are usually reported between ages 18 months and 3 years.)
• tremors
• in infant, floppy extremities that later seem stiff
• lack of movement of one or more extremities
• failure to achieve developmental milestones as compared with other children (This is what often prompts caregivers to seek medical care.)
• unusual posture or crawling movement
• toe walking
• speech problems
• clumsy, uncoordinated movements
• behavioral and personality problems

Objective
• hyperactive deep tendon reflexes (especially with the spastic type)
• scissoring of the legs
• contractures
• atrophy of a limb
• delayed gross motor development
• muscle weakness, dystonia, imbalance, and lack of coordination (most common with the ataxic type)
• mental retardation (in 50% of patients)
• early hand dominance (before the child is age 18 to 24 months)
• persistent infant reflexes
• fisting after age 4 months
• attention deficit disorders.

Nursing diagnosis
Altered Growth and Development related to handicaps associated with brain damage
Desired outcome: Parents and child (if appropriate) demonstrate an understanding of the reason for developmental deficit and impaired mobility and participate in the habituation process.

Interventions
1. Assess the child for the following:
• degree of developmental delay, using the DDST or another appropriate tool
• neurologic dysfunction (using an audiogram, if indicated)
• musculoskeletal deformity or dysfunction.
2. Help the child and his caregivers to maximize the child's developmental potential and to accept the condition.
3. Provide emotional support and help the caregivers to deal with feelings of guilt associated with the disorder.
4. Promote the child's independence in feeding by:
• encouraging use of adaptive utensils (such as double-handled cups, large-handled spoons, fixed straws, and rimmed plates with suction cups)

• preparing finger foods
• providing positive reinforcement.
5. Encourage proper positioning and exercises to prevent contractures and promote comfort.
6. Provide proper care during use of support and immobilization devices, including:
• meticulous skin care for a child in braces or splints
• proper application and alignment of braces and splints
• supervision of a child using a walker or other appliance for mobilization.
7. Provide appropriate play, stimulation, and educational opportunities.
8. Provide preoperative and postoperative nursing care if surgery is planned.
9. Interact and cooperate with other members of the child's therapeutic team, including physical therapists, occupational therapists, speech therapists, play therapists, school liaisons, and community organizations.

Medical diagnosis

The medical diagnosis for cerebral palsy is based on:
• the patient history and physical examination, including a thorough neurologic and musculoskeletal evaluation
• electromyography (measures the electrical potential of muscles)
• developmental, speech, and hearing tests
• EEG
• computed tomography scan to rule out brain tumors or cysts.

Medical treatment

General treatment goals include early recognition and mobilization of the interdisciplinary health care team to promote the child's optimum autonomy and mental health and to prevent complications.

Congenital clubfoot

Clubfoot refers to various rigid deformities of the shape or position (or both) of one or both feet. Approximately 90% of all children with this disorder have the talipes equinovarus type, in which the metatarsals are turned medially with inversion and plantar flexion of the foot.

Occurring in varying degrees among affected children, clubfoot is more common among boys and is often associated with other congenital disorders, such as spina bifida. Suggested etiologies include abnormal intrauterine development or position.

Assessment

Unless the deformity is extremely mild, clubfoot usually is noted at or immediately after birth. The foot cannot be manipulated into a correct position, as can a positional deformity.

Nursing diagnosis

Impaired Physical Mobility related to the effects of the congenital musculoskeletal deformity of clubfoot

Desired outcome: After appropriate therapeutic intervention, the foot assumes correct alignment.

Interventions

1. Assess parental understanding and acceptance of the deformity and treatment plan; provide information and emotional support, as necessary.
2. Promote correction of the foot to the normal position and function by assisting with the selected procedures, including:
• casting in successively corrected positions
• use of a Denis Browne splint
• use of a wedged cast
• manipulation and stretching of the foot before immobilization (*Note:* The final position of immobilization will be overcorrective.)
• surgery involving tendons or bones if conservative measures fail.
3. Prevent the development of complications as with any patient in a cast or splint:
• Monitor the circulation and ennervation of the involved foot by assessing skin color, temperature, sensation, movement, and capillary refill time.
• Position and reposition the child frequently for comfort, mobility, alignment, and prevention of sores, contractures, and cast damage.
• Provide adequate nutrition and hydration.
• Monitor the child's elimination patterns to maintain function and prevent cast soiling.
• Encourage mobility within prescribed limits.
• Provide appropriate skin care.
• Promote a balance between rest and activity.
• Soothe the child and communicate with him.
4. Instruct the caregivers, especially the primary caregiver, in long-term care measures. (Hospitalization usually is short-term for application of casts or splints only.) Such teaching should include:
• demonstration and return demonstration of manipulation procedures
• instruction on cast care
• demonstration of the application and removal of splints or braces
• reinforcement of the doctor's instructions
• instruction on assessing the neurovascular status of the child's extremities (see *Checking neurovascular status*)
• encouragement to frequently hold and comfort the child in spite of the cast or appliance

CHECKING NEUROVASCULAR STATUS

Instruct caregivers to do the following when checking the neurovascular status of a child with a neuromuscular deformity, such as congenital clubfoot:
• Observe the color of the fingers and toes; should not be pale or cyanotic (which indicates circulatory compromise).
• Look for swelling; note the size of the digits.
• Check and compare the temperature of the digits; should be approximately body temperature and uniform from one digit to another.
• Check sensation by touching the extremity and asking the child whether he feels anything.
• Check the child's ability to move the extremity.
• Feel for pulses.
• Check for rapid refilling of the nail beds after compressing them.

• emphasis on the need for frequent follow-up visits to reevaluate the child's status and for an extended maintenance period requiring special shoes or night splints (or both).

Medical diagnosis

Medical diagnosis is based on direct observation, manipulation, and X-ray evaluation.

Medical treatment

The goal is to begin treatment as early as possible to correct the deformity and maintain the correct anatomic position. Conservative therapy is preferred unless the deformity is resistant or a relapse to the former position occurs, in which case surgery may be required.

Congenital hip dysplasia

A malformation of one or both hips, congenital hip dysplasia is classified according to the degree of dysplasia as:
• shallow acetabulum—the mildest form in which the hip is unstable
• subluxation—incomplete dislocation in which the head of the femur rides up and out of the hip socket
• dislocation—displacement of the head of the femur completely out of the acetabulum.

Hip dysplasia, more common among girls than boys, occurs most frequently in breech and cesarean section deliveries. When only one hip is affected, the left hip is usually involved.
Although the etiology is unknown, hereditary, hormonal, and intrauterine factors may be involved.

Nurses working in newborn nurseries are responsibile for recording and reporting the following observations:
• restricted abduction of the hip joint
• unequal leg lengths
• asymmetrical gluteal and thigh folds
• broadness of the perineum.
Note: Some forms of congenital hip dysplasia are not manifested until walking begins.

Assessment

Frequently encountered data for congenital hip dysplasia include the following:

Subjective

• delayed walking
• limping, swaying, or lurching (with toddlers)
• unequal leg lengths (noticed by one pant leg appearing longer than the other)
• swayed back

Objective

• lordosis and potbellied appearance
• unstable gait
• unequal leg lengths
• Trendelenburg gait (pelvis on the normal side droops when the heel of the affected side strikes the floor).

Nursing diagnosis

Impaired Physical Mobility related to the effects of musculoskeletal hip deformity and the therapeutic management of the disorder by casting, splinting, or traction
Desired outcome: The child will walk with an even gait after treatment.

Interventions

1. Implement all measures that apply to managing a child in traction or a cast. (Bryant's traction may be used for bilateral dysplasia.)
2. Provide the caregivers—especially the primary caregiver responsible for maintaining therapy—with teaching and encouragement. Keep in mind that feeding may be a special problem because of the child's positioning.
3. Follow the usual preoperative and postoperative measures for children requiring surgery (see Section 4 for details).

Medical diagnosis

The medical diagnosis for congenital hip dysplasia is based on:
• subjective and objective signs and symptoms
• X-rays (not of much value until later changes occur)
• positive Ortolani's sign (With the child positioned on his back, the knees and hips are flexed with the knees together; then, the legs are slowly abducted 90 degrees. If the hip [or hips] is dislocated, the head of the femur can be felt slipping into the acetabulum with a click when pressure is applied from behind.)
• positive Barlow's sign (Pressure applied anteriorly causes the head of the femur to push out of and over the posterior edge of the acetabulum. Release of pressure causes the head of the femur to return to its previous position.)
• positive Allis' sign. (With the child placed supinely on a hard surface, the knees and hips are flexed. One knee lower than the other in this position indicates unilateral hip dysplasia.)

Medical treatment

Treatment goals include early detection and intervention to correct the deformity.

If hip dysplasia is recognized early, it often is treated by gradual abduction with double diapering. Older children may be treated with a Frejka pillow splint, a Paulington harness, or an abduction brace and are managed on an outpatient basis. Children with severe dysplasia or those with secondary changes in their condition from weight bearing may require hospitalization. The duration of the hospitalization is usally short-term for children requiring application of a cast or brace only; however, those requiring open reduction will require a longer stay.

Down's syndrome

Also known as mongolism and trisomy 21, Down's syndrome is caused by one of the following three possible patterns of chromosomal abnormalities:

• trisomy 21, the most common type, occurs most frequently in children born to older women

• the translocation type, involving translocation of chromosomal material, is unrelated to maternal age but demonstrates a familial tendency

• the mosaic type, the rarest of the three patterns, occurs in children with some abnormal and some normal chromosomal patterns.

Children with Down's syndrome have some degree of mental retardation and the characteristic "Oriental" facies from which the term mongolism derives. They have a high incidence of congenital heart anomalies (such as patent ductus arteriosus, atrial septal defect, and ventricular septal defect) and an incidence of chronic myelogenous leukemia 20 times greater than in the general population, as well as other chronic medical problems that put them at high risk for frequent hospitalization.

Assessment

Frequently encountered data in a Down's syndrome child admitted to the pediatric unit may include the following (as well as the usual clinical signs listed under "Medical diagnosis"):

Subjective

• frequent urinary tract infections

• visual defects

• earaches

• feeding problems (sucks or eats poorly)

• bowel problems (prone to constipation)

(*Note:* The subjective complaints listed above will vary depending on the reason for admission to the hospital. Be sure to obtain information on feeding, toileting, and medicating techniques at the time of admission.)

Objective
• poor muscle tone
• cardiac murmurs and dysrhythmias
• characteristic mongoloid facies
• crackles and rhonchi
• infected bulging tympanic membranes
• nasal discharge
• delayed developmental level
• conjunctivitis
• elevated temperature.

Nursing diagnosis
Ineffective Airway Clearance related to decreased muscle tone, mouth breathing, or nasal congestion (specify)
Desired outcome: The child has no signs of choking or airway obstruction.

Interventions
1. Monitor the child for signs and symptoms of:
• respiratory infection, ineffective airway clearance, or both
• temperature elevation
• dyspnea or tachypnea
• tachycardia.
2. Promote drainage and decrease secretions.
3. Provide humidification with a cool mist vaporizer.
4. Reposition the child frequently.
5. Perform chest physiotherapy, as ordered.
6. Assist the child with incentive spirometry.
7. Administer bronchodilators, mucolytics, and antibiotics, as ordered.

Nursing diagnosis
Altered Nutrition: Less Than Body Requirements related to feeding problems and GI disorders
Desired outcome: The child receives nutrition adequate for the needs of surgery, growth, and healing.

Interventions
1. Provide small, frequent feedings.
2. Aspirate the child's nose with a bulb syringe before feedings.
3. Increase the child's fluid and roughage intake to prevent constipation.
4. During feeding, maintain the child in an upright position with support, as necessary.
5. Provide finger foods appropriate for the child's developmental level.
6. Provide large-handled utensils.
7. During feeding, make sure that food is pushed back past the child's large, protuberant tongue.

Nursing diagnosis

Self-care Deficit (specify) related to delayed development
Desired outcome: The child uses self-help skills.

Interventions

1. Set realistic short-term goals.
2. Involve the child and caregivers in an exercise program.
3. Involve the child and caregivers in a stimulation program.
4. Teach the child skills in short, repetitive sessions.
5. Praise the child frequently for his efforts.
6. Provide continuous evaluation of the child's progress, and revise goals as necessary.

Nursing diagnosis

Altered Cardiac Output, Decreased: Fatigue related to tissue hypoxia secondary to cardiac anomaly
(For information on the desired outcome and specific interventions, see "Congenital heart defects" under the "Cardiovascular and respiratory systems" heading in this section.)

Medical diagnosis

The medical diagnosis for Down's syndrome is based on:
• amniocentesis studies (to detect the disorder in utero)
• family history or maternal age (may lead to suspicion about the disorder)
• clinical signs, including:
  —simean crease
  —flat nasal bridge
  —low-set ears
  —large, protruding tongue
  —hypotonic muscles
  —flat occiput
  —oblique palpable fissures
  —delayed development
• chromosomal studies.

Medical treatment

General treatment goals include:
• prompt diagnosis
• early treatment, including:
  —short-term therapy (preventing physical problems)
  —long-term therapy (promoting maximum development by beginning treatment early in infancy)
• genetic counseling.
  Specific goals are related to presenting signs and symptoms.

Fracture

A break in the continuity of a bone, a fracture is usually classified according to the bone tissue involved and the nature of the break. Although a childhood fracture is a traumatic condition that may require hospitalization, the fracture tends to heal quite rapidly because of the active osteogenic potential of the child's bone. In fact, the younger the child, the faster the bone will heal. Unless the fracture is complicated, the child probably will be hospitalized for only a short period.

Because of his incomplete gross motor development and the types of activity in which he participates, a child is more likely than an adult to sustain a fracture. The most common fracture sustained during childhood is of the clavicle. Fracture of the femur is common among school-age children who are struck by automobiles (at this age, the child's femur is approximately at the same level as the bumper).

Fractures in infants may be the result of abuse, neglect, or careless handling and should be treated as suspect. Multiple fractures in various stages of healing are suspicious in any child.

Because a child's bones are more porous and flexible than those of an adult, fractures may be of a different type (such as a greenstick fracture, in which one side of the bone is broken while the other side is bent). A child's bones may even sustain severe bending without fracturing; however, such bending may result in a curved-type deformity.

Children are at particular risk for damage to the cartilaginous epiphyseal plate, which could result in growth deformities. To prevent such complications, fractures in this area are frequently managed by open reduction and internal fixation.

Assessment
Frequently encountered data for fractures include the following:
Subjective
• pain (may be minimal in a greenstick fracture)
• refusal to walk (usually occurs with a small child)

Objective
(The following signs may be only minimally evident in a greenstick fracture.)
• inability to move the affected body part
• ecchymosis
• edema
• deformity
• decreased range of motion
• crepitus
• guarding.

Nursing diagnosis
Impaired Physical Mobility: Limited Range of Motion related to bone fracture and therapeutic immobilization
Desired outcome: The fracture is reduced; the position, maintained; and the function, restored.

Interventions
1. Institute comfort measures for the child who is in traction or a cast.
2. Provide care for the child in traction or a cast similar to care measures for an adult; however, keep in mind that fecal and urine contamination will be a greater threat.
3. Institute preoperative and postoperative care if open reduction is required.
4. Encourage and provide diversional activities, including:
• entertainment
• toys (However, keep in mind that children are likely to place small toys or other objects in a cast.)
• environmental changes (such as walking the child in a stroller or wheeling the child around in a wagon).

Nursing diagnosis
Altered Comfort: Acute Pain related to bone fracture
Desired outcome: The child's pain is relieved or reduced.

Interventions
1. Position the child for comfort and alignment.
2. Give analgesics, as needed and ordered.
3. Provide emotional support.
4. Institute safety precautions to avoid complications or further trauma.

Medical diagnosis
The medical diagnosis for fractures is based on:
• clinical signs
• X-rays.

Medical treatment
Treatment includes reduction and immobilization.

Hydrocephalus
Hydrocephalus is the excessive accumulation of fluid within the cranial vault leading to dilatation of the ventricles, increased intracranial pressure (ICP), and brain compression. Caused by an imbalance between the production and absorption (or obstruction of pathways) of cerebrospinal fluid (CSF), this condition may be congenital or acquired as a result of trauma or disease.
    Hydrocephalus is categorized as follows:
• noncommunicating—caused by an obstruction in CSF flow
• communicating—caused by faulty absorption of CSF
• hypersecretory—caused by excessive CSF secretion.
    Congenital hydrocephalus may be associated with other anomalies.

Assessment
Frequently encountered data for hydrocephalus include the following:

Subjective
- listlessness
- irritability
- loss of appetite
- shrill cry
- headache
- nausea or vomiting (or both)
- personality changes
- incontinence
- difficulty walking
- impaired mental functioning
- diplopia or blurred vision

Objective
- in infant, enlargement of the head by more than ⅜″ (1 cm) in 2 weeks
- separation of the sutures
- bulging fontanelles
- dilation of the scalp veins
- Macewen's sign ("cracked pot" percussion)
- persistent infant reflexes
- seizures
- opisthotonos.

Nursing diagnosis
Potential for Injury: Aspiration, Falls, or Decubitus Ulcers (specify) related to effects of neurologic deficit
Desired outcome: No injuries (such as aspiration, falls, or decubitus ulcers) occur.

Interventions
1. Take the following precautions to prevent aspiration:
- Assess the child's gag and swallow reflexes before feeding.
- Offer food slowly in small amounts.
- Position the child on his side after feeding.
- Keep suction equipment available in the child's room.
2. Take the following measures to prevent skin breakdown:
- Turn the child every 2 hours (check doctor's orders for permissible head positions).
- Keep the child's skin clean and dry.
- Provide adequate nutrition.
- Monitor pressure points.
- Provide a special surface area under the child's head, such as an alternating pressure mattress.
3. To prevent neck trauma, support the child's head when lifting, moving, and turning him; be sure to rotate the head with the body.
4. Because hydrocephalus may cause gait disturbances in an ambulatory child, take the following measures to prevent falls:
- Identify and remove potential hazards from the child's room or pathway.

• Supervise the child's ambulation and activities.
5. Take necessary seizure precautions.

Nursing diagnosis

Potential for Infection related to effects of surgical procedure to shunt CSF
Desired outcome: The child remains free of infection.

Interventions (postoperative)

1. Monitor and report signs or symptoms of possible meningitis, peritonitis, or septicemia, including:
• fever
• nuchal rigidity
• Kernig's sign
• Brudzinski's sign
• headache
• photophobia
• abdominal tenderness or rigidity (or both)
• signs of increased ICP, including:
— change in level of consciousness or behavior (or both)
— headache
— increased systolic blood pressure
— widening pulse pressure
— bradycardia or bradypnea
— increased head circumference (during infancy)
— projectile vomiting.
2. Monitor the child's wounds for possible infection; report any of the following signs or symptoms:
• redness
• drainage
• edema
• tenderness.
3. Take the following measures to prevent infection:
• Use strict aseptic technique for all dressing changes and other procedures.
• Keep wound areas clean and dry.
• Administer antibiotics, as ordered.

Nursing diagnosis

Altered Parenting related to interruption of the bonding process secondary to illness and hospitalization
Desired outcome: The caregivers are attentive and loving toward their child, showing appropriate caregiving behaviors.

Interventions

1. Provide a permissive visiting atmosphere.
2. Encourage touching and holding.
3. Encourage age-appropriate stimulation.
4. Include the caregivers in care activities.
5. Recognize the stages of grief and encourage the caregivers to verbalize their feelings.

Nursing diagnosis

Knowledge Deficit related to lack of previous exposure to or experience with hydrocephalus

Desired outcome: The caregivers and child (if appropriate) demonstrate an understanding of hydrocephalus and the plan of treatment.

Interventions

1. Answer questions simply, honestly, and as completely as possible based on the family's capacity to understand.
2. Be prepared to offer information on resources (brochures, booklets).
3. Teach about possible shunt problems, such as clogging, kinking, separation, or valve insufficiency.
4. Explain all procedures.
5. Teach the child and family preoperatively and postoperatively.
6. Teach the family which signs and symptoms of complications (such as shunt failure, increased ICP, infection, and dehydration) to report to the doctor.
7. Teach the caregivers how to pump the shunt, if appropriate.
8. Refer the caregivers to local social agencies or parent support groups.

Medical diagnosis

The medical diagnosis for hydrocephalus is based on:
• the physical examination and patient history, including serial head measurements
• computed tomography or brain scan
• skull X-rays
• ventriculography
• transillumination
• cerebral angiography
• ultrasonography.

Medical treatment

Using a multidisciplinary approach, treatment aims to correct the underlying cause, if possible, before extensive cortical atrophy occurs. Treatment may include:
• removal of a tumor, cyst, or mass (if present)
• widening of the foramen magnum
• shunting (usually to the right atrium of the heart or to the peritoneal cavity) to bypass an obstruction that cannot be removed
• maximum habilitation for independent living within the limits imposed by neurologic and intellectual damage (if associated with other anomalies, such as myelomeningocele, prognosis may be poor)
• anticonvulsants to control seizures
• occasional use of drugs, such as acetazolamide, to reduce CSF production (success has been limited with this therapy).

Meningitis

An inflammation or infection of the membranes that cover the brain and spinal cord, meningitis may be caused by bacteria, viruses, parasites, fungi, or irritation from a tumor or chemical. Peak incidence occurs between ages 3 months and 3 years. The organism most commonly responsible is *Hemophilus influenzae,* which abounds among day-care populations. In infants younger than age 3 months, the primary causative organisms are Group B streptococci and *Escherichia coli.*

Before the advent of effective antimicrobial agents, the mortality for bacterial meningitis was between 50% and 90%. Even today, survivors may suffer long-term sequelae.

The usual infiltrative route of bacterial meningitis is via the upper respiratory tract into the bloodstream (bacteremia), then to the vascular supply of the meninges. Otitis media may lead to meningitis via direct extension. Any trauma that interrupts the integrity of the skull can result in the introduction of organisms into the meninges. Other possible routes include the skin and genitourinary tract. There, bacteria multiply, enter the bloodstream, and eventually penetrate the blood-brain barrier.

Assessment

Signs and symptoms of meningitis depend greatly on the child's age and the causative organism. Frequently encountered data include the following:

Subjective
• history of upper respiratory tract infection, otitis media, or GI disorder
• convulsive movements
• fever
• photophobia
• headache
• stiff neck
• vomiting
• anorexia
• irritability

Objective
(Some of the following symptoms are extremely vague in newborns.)
• projectile vomiting and other signs of increased intracranial pressure (ICP)
• opisthotonos
• paradoxical irritability
• in infant, tense fontanelle (usually a late sign)
• positive Brudzinski's sign
• positive Kernig's sign.

Nursing diagnosis

Potential for Injury related to loss of motor control secondary to seizures

Desired outcome: Patient safety is maintained and seizures are prevented through observation and compliance with treatment regimen.

Interventions

1. Once the child is hospitalized (should be immediately after diagnosis is made), institute infection control precautions.
2. Take a baseline neurologic assessment.
3. Monitor for signs and symptoms of:
• increased ICP (see the interventions for "Hydrocephalus" in this section for a complete list)
• bulging fontanelles
• Macewen's sign
• irritability
• high-pitched cry.
4. If ICP monitoring is used, assist with placement of a monitoring device (if this is done on the unit). Provide perioperative care if the procedure requires surgical intervention. Monitor and record pressure readings after insertion of devices (see *Three ways to monitor intracranial pressure,* page 72). Report significant changes immediately.
5. Assist with diagnostic studies and expedite the handling of specimens.
6. Take necessary seizure precautions, because increased ICP may result in seizures (see "Seizure disorders" in this section for additional interventions).
7. Monitor for signs of increased cerebral edema, which may result in inappropriate secretion of antidiuretic hormone associated with meningitis. Maintain careful intake and output records.
8. Minimize external stimuli, such as lights, noise, and activity.
9. Administer medications (including antibiotics and anticonvulsants) promptly, as ordered.
10. Monitor and control fever to prevent seizures.
11. Maintain I.V. access.

Nursing diagnosis

Altered Thought Processes related to the effects of central nervous system tissue destruction or fever

Desired outcome: The child has no neurologic deficit and returns to his preillness level of functioning.

Interventions

1. Perform neurologic checks every 2 hours.
2. Monitor fluid intake and output and electrolyte balance.
3. Provide continuous reality orientation.
4. Take measures to control fever.

5. Monitor respiratory status (hypoxia will elevate already increased ICP and cause further damage).

Nursing diagnosis

Altered Comfort: Pain related to acute headache and photophobia secondary to meningeal irritation, increased ICP, or both
Desired outcome: Child is free of pain or has minimal discomfort.

Interventions
1. Elevate the head of the bed 30 degrees.
2. Keep the room quiet and dimly lit.
3. Administer analgesics, as ordered.
4. Avoid jostling or startling the child.
5. Control the number and noise level of visitors.
6. Avoid excessive handling of an infant with meningitis.

Nursing diagnosis

Potential for Sensory-Perceptual Alteration: Auditory deficit related to delay in treatment or ototoxic properties of medications
Desired outcome: The child has no evidence of hearing loss or, if hearing loss is detected, receives early intervention to prevent delays in language development or intellectual deprivation.

Interventions
Encourage follow-up audiograms for a child who is receiving long-term or high-dose aminoglycoside therapy.

Nursing diagnosis

Knowledge Deficit related to lack of information on disease etiology, treatment, and communicability
Desired outcome: The caregivers and child (if appropriate) verbalize an understanding of the nature of the disease and thereby prevent spreading the disease.

Interventions
1. Assess the caregivers' and child's knowledge level and correct any misconceptions they may have.
2. Discuss the possibility of infection of the child's contacts.
3. Encourage the use of prophylactic medications, such as rifampin, or vaccines for persons who have had close contact with the child.
4. Review with the caregivers the factors responsibile for the child's susceptibility to the disease.
5. Discuss discharge plans and follow-up visits.
6. Clarify any doctor's instructions.

Medical diagnosis

The medical diagnosis for meningitis is based on:
• an adequate patient history and physical examination (essential)
• septic workup (for early identification of responsible organisms), including:
    —lumbar puncture

—blood cultures
—complete blood count
—urinalysis.

Medical treatment
Treatment includes:
• aggressive antimicrobial therapy
• symptomatic and supportive therapy if meningitis is aseptic (viral) (Viral meningitis is usually benign and self-limiting.)
• maintenance of cardiopulmonary status
• seizure prevention
• administration of anticonvulsants
• administration of antibiotics (Antibiotics with known risks for serious adverse reactions may also be used because of the life-threatening nature of meningitis.)
• administration of rifampin prophylactically to contacts.

Reye's syndrome
An acute, often fatal, hepatic encephalopathy affecting children (primarily school-age children) and adolescents, Reye's syndrome may occur after a mild infection, such as chicken pox, flu, or Epstein-Barr infection. It is attributed to liver failure in the conversion of ammonia to urea, resulting in toxic blood levels.

Recently, researchers have linked Reye's syndrome with the use of aspirin in the management of a prodromal viral infection. In 1982, the Committee on Infectious Diseases issued a caution on the use of aspirin for children with viral infections.

Assessment
Signs and symptoms of Reye's syndrome depend on the disease stage.

Stage I
(The following subjective symptoms usually prompt the caregivers to seek medical attention for the child.)
• lethargy and fatigue
• behavioral changes
• vomiting
(*Note:* Beyond Stage I, manifestations are mainly objective.)

Stage II
• hyperreactive reflexes
• combative behavior
• stupor
• delirium
• hepatomegaly and abnormal liver function test results
• abnormal EEG reading
• hypoglycemia
• rash

Stage III
• coma
• decorticate rigidity
• hyperventilation
• nonreactive pupils

Stage IV
• deep coma
• fixed pupils
• decerebrate rigidity

Stage V
• flaccidity
• absent deep tendon reflexes
• seizures
• respiratory arrest.

Nursing diagnosis
Altered Thought Processes related to hypoglycemia, elevated
serum ammonia levels, and cerebral edema
Desired outcome: The child has no edema and maintains normal
ammonia and blood glucose levels throughout hospitalization.

Interventions
1. Perform an ongoing assessment of the child's mental status
and behavioral changes. (If possible, one nurse should be assigned consistently so that subtle changes can be noted.)
2. Assist with continuous intracranial pressure (ICP) monitoring,
if instituted (see *Three ways to monitor intracranial pressure,*
page 72).
3. Provide a low-protein diet; compensate for calorie deficiencies
with additional carbohydrates.
4. Maintain I.V. lines.
5. Monitor the child's fluid intake and output for signs and symptoms of dehydration or fluid retention.
6. Provide adequate hydration but avoid overhydration. (I.V.
fluids may include dextrose 10% with insulin.)
7. Assist with obtaining laboratory specimens.
8. Monitor the following laboratory values:
• electrolyte levels
• blood glucose levels
• ammonia levels
• liver enzyme studies.
9. Promote bowel management by administering:
• stool softeners, as ordered, to prevent constipation
• enteric bactericides (such as kanamycin and neomycin), as ordered, to decrease intestinal ammonia production.
10. As ordered, use the following measures to promote diarrhea
and remove protein from the intestine:
• enemas

THREE WAYS TO MONITOR INTRACRANIAL PRESSURE

Elevated intracranial pressure (ICP) may cause life-threatening complications in central nervous system infections. Here are three ICP surveillance methods:

Ventricular catheter monitoring, the most direct and accurate method, permits evaluation of brain compliance and drainage of large amounts of cerebrospinal fluid (CSF). It also carries the greatest risk of infection. A small rubber catheter enters the lateral ventricle through a burr hole, and its fluid-filled line connects to a domed transducer and a display monitor. If ICP is elevated, pressure ex-dome's diaphragm.

Subarachnoid screw monitoring carries less risk of infection and tissue damage because the screw doesn't penetrate the cerebrum. Instead, it enters the subarachnoid space, then connects to a transducer as in ventricular catheter monitoring.

Epidural sensor monitoring, the least invasive method with the lowest risk of infection, provides questionable accuracy because it doesn't measure ICP directly from a CSF-filled space. Instead, it uses a fiber-optic sensor placed in the epidural space, with cable connection to a monitor.

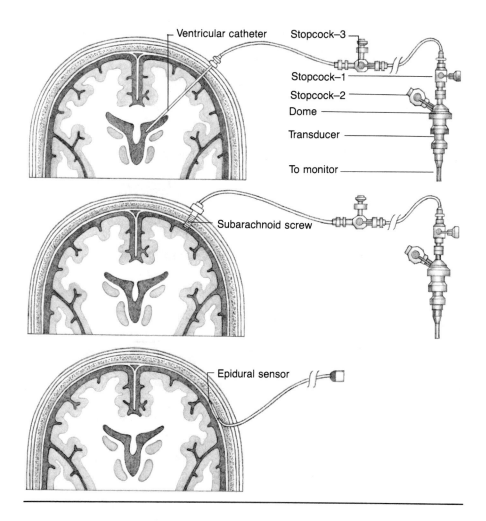

• lactulose
• magnesium sulfate.
11. Administer mannitol or other medications, as ordered, to decrease cerebral edema.
12. Provide reality orientation in cooperation with the child's caregivers; encourage them to bring in familiar items from home.

Nursing diagnosis
Potential for Injury related to mental confusion or loss of motor control secondary to seizures (or both)
Desired outcome: The child has no evidence of mental confusion, seizures, or their resulting injuries.

Interventions
1. Provide close supervision.
2. Take necessary seizure precautions (see "Seizure disorders" in this section for details).
3. Take measures to control fever, including the possible use of a hypothermia blanket.

Nursing diagnosis
Potential Fluid Volume Deficit related to bleeding secondary to decreased production of clotting factors by the liver
Desired outcome: The child has no evidence of bleeding throughout the hospitalization.

Interventions
1. Use the smallest-gauge needle available for all injections.
2. Apply direct pressure to all puncture sites until bleeding has stopped.
3. Observe for and report blood in the child's urine and stool (may require testing for occult blood).
4. Observe the child's gums and mucous membranes for trauma or bleeding; avoid abrasive oral hygiene measures, such as flossing.
5. Monitor results of coagulation studies.
6. Administer vitamins K and B complex, as ordered.

Nursing diagnosis
Ineffective Breathing Pattern related to debilitated state, central nervous system involvement, or pancuronium bromide treatment (specify)
Desired outcome: The child has normal respiratory function and arterial blood gas levels throughout the hospitalization.

Interventions
1. Monitor respiratory status, including respiratory rate, rhythm, and depth as well as lung sounds.
2. Monitor arterial blood gas levels and pulse oximetry results.
3. Be prepared to assist with emergency endotracheal intubation, if required.
4. Be prepared to assist with mechanical ventilation, if necessary

(because hypoventilation increases ICP).
5. Provide emotional support to prevent hyperventilation.

Nursing diagnosis

Powerlessness related to overwhelming illness and intimidation by the hospital environment
Desired outcome: The child verbalizes a sense of control and has no complications induced by emotional stress.

Interventions

1. Explain all equipment and procedures to the caregivers and child.
2. Give the child choices (with meals, activities, and forms of medication) whenever possible.
3. Provide continuity of care to build rapport.
4. If the child is comatose, provide care as if he could see and hear.
5. Keep the caregivers informed of the child's activities and progress so that they can act as liaisons for family, friends, and school.
Remember: In pediatrics, the patient is the family. The diagnosis of powerlessness extends to the caregivers as well. Refer them to the National Reye's Syndrome Foundation, P.O. Box R.S., Benzonia, Mich. 49616, for additional support.

Medical diagnosis

The medical diagnosis for Reye's syndrome is based on:
• history of recent viral infection
• clinical signs and symptoms
• laboratory findings, including:
  —abnormal liver function studies (elevated serum glutamic oxaloacetic transaminase and serum glutamic pyruvic transaminase levels and prolonged prothrombin time)
  —low blood glucose levels
  —elevated serum ammonia levels.

Medical treatment

Treatment should be supportive. Goals include:
• reducing cerebral edema
• maintaining acid-base balance
• maintaining blood glucose levels
• supporting vital functions.
  Initial efforts, including those listed under the interventions above, will be conservative. However, if conservative measures fail, treatment may include:
• peritoneal dialysis to reduce blood ammonia levels
• exchange transfusions to temporarily remove toxins
• craniectomy to relieve ICP

• curarization to reduce ICP
• barbiturate-induced coma to reduce cerebral metabolic requirements.

Scoliosis

A common childhood deformity characterized by lateral curvature and rotation of the spine, scoliosis is seen most often in adolescent girls during the growth spurt. Most cases of scoliosis are idiopathic; however, the deformity also is associated with infectious and paralytic diseases. A familial tendency has been demonstrated.

Scoliosis is classified as either functional or structural. Functional scoliosis may be transient from muscle spasm or nerve root compression; it also may be postural, correctable by proper positioning. Structural scoliosis is inflexible and not correctable by positioning.

Assessment

Frequently encountered data for scoliosis include the following:

Subjective

Scoliosis is asymptomatic unless severe, in which case the symptoms include:
• GI symptoms (from crowding of the abdominal organs), including heartburn, flatulence, cramps, and indigestion
• respiratory symptoms (from diminished respiratory capacity), including poor exercise tolerance and proneness to respiratory infections.

Minor deformity may be discovered during routine physicals, sports examinations, or school scoliosis screenings. Caregivers may overlook the deformity because adolescents are reticent about undressing in their presence. However, caregivers may notice that the child's hemlines or pant legs are uneven.

Objective

• "C" or "S" curvature of the spine
• prominence of one hip or scapula (or both the hip and scapula)
• difference in shoulder height
• rib cage deformity
• rib hump noted when child bends forward.

Nursing diagnosis

Disturbance in Self-concept: Body Image and Self-esteem related to effects of spinal deformity distinguishing adolescent from peers
Desired outcome: The child verbalizes positive body image, self-esteem, and optimism concerning treatment outcome.

Interventions

1. Explain all procedures and appliances used in treatment.
2. Give special attention to the psychological aspects of the treat-

ment. For example, be an active listener and allow the child time to voice his concerns. Also, establish a channel for open communication of fears, and help the child to recognize positive self-concepts.

3. Encourage personal grooming.

4. Focus on the positive outcome of treatment.

Nursing diagnosis

Anxiety related to threat of physical pain, loss of mobility, or both

Desired outcome: The child verbalizes anxieties and seeks information or resources to deal with them.

Interventions

1. Assess the child's level of understanding and ease at verbalizing his feelings.

2. Discuss pain management with the child and his caregivers.

3. Develop a rapport and open communication with the child and his caregivers.

4. Help to develop alternative methods of mobility.

5. Permit as much independence as possible.

6. Explore with the child and his caregivers avenues of socialization during treatment, including telephoning or writing friends, visiting with relatives and friends, participating in activities (as tolerated), and working on homework assignments with peers.

7. Encourage the child's attendance at school.

Nursing diagnosis

Impaired Skin Integrity related to appliances used in treating scoliosis

Desired outcome: Skin integrity remains intact throughout the use of casts or braces.

Interventions

1. Provide nursing care for the child in a cast or traction.

2. Assess the child's brace for proper fit.

3. Investigate all of the child's complaints without delay.

4. Assess the skin for irritation.

5. Teach the child and family members to observe and report signs of skin breakdown during home treatment.

Nursing diagnosis

Potential for Injury: Neurovascular Trauma related to pressure from corrective appliance

Desired outcome: The child's neurovascular status proximal and distal to the appliance is normal.

Interventions

1. Monitor and report any color, temperature, sensation, or movement variations.

2. Monitor the child's peripheral pulses.

Medical diagnosis

The medical diagnosis for scoliosis is based on:
• physical assessment findings
• spinal and chest X-rays.

Medical treatment

The goal is to correct the lateral and rotational deformities and to maintain the correction until growth is complete. Various approaches may be used, depending on the nature and degree of deformity, including:
• management of curves of 40 degrees or less by exercise or electrical stimulation (on an outpatient basis)
• braces, such as the Milwaukee brace and molded plastic jacket
• spinal fusion with instrumentation or internal fixation.

Seizure disorders

Common childhood neurologic dysfunctions involving abnormal electical activity of the brain, seizure disorders produce a myriad of symptoms depending on the site of the activity in the central nervous system. For an explanation of specific types of seizures, see *Understanding seizures,* pages 78 and 79.

Although hospitalization usually is not required for children with seizure disorders, it may be necessary if the seizures are of recent origin and a diagnostic workup is indicated, or if status epilepticus is involved. However, any hospitalized child with a history of seizures must be carefully monitored because physical or psychological stress can lower the seizure threshold.

Status epilepticus, considered a medical emergency, involves a rapid succession of seizures without intervening periods of recovery or one continuous seizure lasting longer than 30 minutes. It may result from failure to take anticonvulsant medications, hypoglycemia, high fever, poisoning, head injury, brain tumor, infection, or drug or alcohol use or sudden withdrawal. If unarrested, this seizure type can cause cerebral hypoxia, resulting in irreversible brain damage or death.

Assessment

Status epilepticus. If the child is admitted to the hospital for status epilepticus, defer assessment and institute the following emergency measures:
• Establish and maintain an airway for respiratory functioning.
  —Assist with intubation, if needed.
  —Suction, as needed.
• Administer oxygen, as needed and ordered.
• Institute assisted ventilation, if needed.
• Establish an I.V. line to:

UNDERSTANDING SEIZURES

When we talk about a seizure, we're referring to abnormal electrical discharges from the brain's neurons. And, depending on the location and number of these discharges, a seizure may cause unconsciousness, convulsive movements, or motor, sensory, or behavioral abnormalities.

In children, the risk of seizure is greatest between birth and age 2; between ages 5 and 7; and at the onset of puberty, when girls are at greater risk than boys.

As you probably know, recurring seizures, called epilepsy, are divided into two groups: partial (electrical discharges occur in a localized area of the brain) and generalized (discharges occur simultaneously in both brain hemispheres). In some patients, partial seizure activity may develop into a generalized seizure.

Within these groups, several specific seizure types exist. The following information will familiarize you with these types. But remember, your patient may exhibit a seizure that deviates from the standard descriptions, or he may experience several seizure types simultaneously.

Partial seizures
• **Simple partial seizures** may have motor or sensory components, depending on discharge location. *Focal sensory seizures* produce tingling, numbness, or warmth in a body part; or visual, auditory, olfactory, or taste disturbances. *Focal motor seizures* produce tonic (muscle stiffening) and clonic (rapid alternate muscle contraction and relaxation) movements of a body part, such as the face, arm, leg, or thumb. In some cases, partial motor seizures spread, and may include one entire side of the body. (These are sometimes called jacksonian seizures.) They may also immediately precede a general tonic-clonic seizure (grand mal seizure).

• **Complex partial seizures,** sometimes called temporal lobe or psychomotor seizures, are characterized by 1- to 2-minute periods when the patient appears to be staring or daydreaming with rapidly fluttering eyelids. He may fall to the ground. In addition, the seizures may produce automatism (repetition of inappropriate acts) such as lip smacking, chewing, and running in circles. Postictal (postseizure) confusion may accompany the staring episodes.

Generalized seizures
• **Absence seizures** (petit mal or lapse seizures) produce brief (10- to 30-second) lapses of awareness. Like complex partial seizures, they make the patient appear to be staring or daydreaming. Although the patient's eyelids flutter rapidly, he doesn't fall or experience automatisms or postictal confusion. He'll resume normal activity without being aware of the attack. Some patients experience 10 or more seizures a day.

—administer anticonvulsants (such as diazepam, phenytoin, phenobarbital, or another barbiturate drip)
   —administer glucose
   —supply fluid and electrolytes.
• Implement safety measures.
• Monitor carefully for cardiac dysrhythmias or signs of respiratory distress.
• Assist during administration of a general anesthetic, as ordered, if seizures do not respond to the measures listed above.
• After establishing control, obtain information regarding the onset and progression of the episode.

Seizure history but no immediate distress. If a child with a history of seizures is admitted to the hospital, obtain the following data:

Subjective
• medications taken for seizures
• age at onset of seizures and the suspected cause

• **Myoclonic seizures** are characterized by brief involuntary muscular jerks of the body or extremities, which may occur rhythmically.

• **Infantile spasms** develop before the child reaches age 1. The seizures produce sudden brief muscle spasms which may affect one part of the body, such as an arm or leg, or affect the body symmetrically. All but 10% of affected infants suffer mental retardation.

• **Akinetic seizures,** or drop attacks, result from a sudden loss of muscle tone. The patient loses consciousness and may fall to the ground. But some patients exhibit only head nodding that lasts just a few seconds.

• **Generalized tonic-clonic (grand mal) seizures** begin abruptly and last several minutes. Moments before the seizure begins, many patients experience an aura or prodrome, such as a change in mood, confusion, a dreamy or floating sensation, visual or taste disturbances, a distinctive smell (such as the odor of orange or a fruity flower), or GI distress. The seizure may begin with a loud cry caused by air rushing from the lungs through the vocal cords. It produces loss of consciousness and causes the patient to fall to the ground. In addition, it produces opisthotonos (arched back) and tonic and clonic movements of all extremities. Other possible effects include incontinence, increased pharyngeal secretions, tongue biting, tachycardia, and hypertension. During the tonic phase, the patient may experience alterations in his breathing pattern, develop cyanosis, and roll his eyes upward. Afterward, he may complain of a headache, exhaustion, or confusion, but he won't remember the seizure. Although this type of seizure is frightening to witness, the child usually doesn't suffer any permanent damage.

Status epilepticus
Status epilepticus is a continuous seizure state in which seizures occur in rapid succession without the patient regaining consciousness between them. Although this condition may be seen with any seizure type, it's usually associated with major motor tonic-clonic seizures. A continuous tonic-clonic seizure is an acute medical emergency and must be stopped immediately before cerebral hypoxia causes irreversible brain damage.

Febrile convulsions
Febrile convulsions aren't usually associated with epilepsy. They may be inherited and usually occur between age 6 months and 3 years. They rarely occur after age 7. The convulsions usually occur in a previously well patient whose temperature suddenly rises to at least 102° F. (38.9° C.). They may produce seizurelike tonic-clonic movements that last less than 10 minutes. Most febrile convulsions are generalized, although some have only partial effects.

• frequency of seizures
• date of last seizure
• description of seizures, including:
  —precipitating factors
  —type of aura, if any
  —where seizures start
  —progression of seizures
  —duration of seizures
  —episodes of incontinence
  —type of movements accompanying seizures
  —status after seizures occur

Objective
• baseline neurologic assessment.

Nursing diagnosis
Potential for Injury related to loss of muscle control and consciousness secondary to seizure

Desired outcome: The child sustains no injuries with seizure activities.

Interventions

1. Take the following measures to help prevent seizure episodes:
• Administer anticonvulsant medications, as ordered.
• Monitor the child's blood drug levels and observe for adverse reactions.
• Identify any precipitating factors and take measures to prevent or minimize the child's exposure to them.
• Keep the bed side rails padded and upright.
• Keep an oral airway device in the child's room.
• Have suction equipment readily available.
• Remove any potential hazards, such as dangerous objects and furniture with sharp edges, from the child's room.
2. If a seizure occurs, protect and observe the child as follows:
• Stay with the child.
• Guide him to the floor if he is out of bed.
• Avoid restraining him; instead, guide his movements.
• Do not force clenched jaws open.
• Turn him onto his side.
• Do not force an object between his teeth.
• Suction as needed.
• Observe and record the following:
　—any aura he experiences
　—the origin and progress of muscle activity
　—episodes of incontinence
　—the chronology of events.

Nursing diagnosis

Ineffective Airway Clearance related to accumulation of secretions during seizure activity
Desired outcome: The child's airway remains patent and no cerebral hypoxia occurs.

Interventions

1. Turn the child onto his side and suction, as needed.
2. Monitor respirations for signs of tachypnea, dyspnea, and apnea; observe for cyanosis.
3. Insert an oral or nasal airway.
4. Monitor arterial blood gas levels, if needed.
5. Administer oxygen, as needed and ordered.
6. Ventilate the child with an Ambu bag if he is apneic.

Nursing diagnosis

Knowledge Deficit related to seizure disorder management
Desired outcome: The caregivers and child (if appropriate) verbalize an understanding of the disorder and participate effectively in the plan of care.

Interventions

1. Provide information about seizure disorders, including a list of possible precipitating factors and how to identify them.
2. Help the child to identify the type of aura he experiences.
3. Explain to the child's caregivers what specific observations should be noted during a seizure episode.
4. Teach the caregivers and child to prepare for seizure activities, including precautions to take for incontinence episodes, tongue biting, and muscle activity. Explain what specific care measures to take during seizure activity.
5. Provide necessary information on anticonvulsant medications, including their possible adverse effects. Offer reassurance that addiction will not occur with long-term treatment.
6. Encourage follow-up visits for monitoring blood levels of medications.
7. Offer instruction on a ketogenic diet, if applicable.
8. Answer any questions the caregivers or child may have and dispel any misconceptions. Refer them to the Epilepsy Foundation of America, 1828 L Street, N.W., Suite 406, Washington, D.C. 20036 for further information.

Nursing diagnosis

Disturbance in Self-concept: Decreased Self-esteem related to diagnosis of seizure disorder and perceived stigma
Desired outcome: The caregivers and child (if applicable) verbalize positive attitudes and maintain as normal a life-style as possible.

Interventions

1. Help the caregivers and child to work through feelings of guilt, anger, and helplessness.
2. Explain about social stigmas and how to manage them.
3. Encourage the caregivers to maintain levels of discipline and to avoid overprotecting the child.
4. Explain that although the disorder will not prevent the child from attending school, the child's teacher needs to be informed about the disorder.
5. Refer the caregivers to counseling or parent support groups, if needed.

Medical diagnosis

The medical diagnosis for seizure disorders is based on:
• the patient history and neurologic assessment
• EEG readings (hyperventilation or photostimulation may be used during the EEG to provoke seizure activity)
• lumbar puncture (to rule out meningitis or subarachnoid hemorrhage)
• computed tomography (to evaluate the ventricles and detect possible tumors)

• cerebral arteriography (to detect vascular abnormalities)
• nurses' observations of the child's seizure activity.

Medical treatment
Treatment for seizure disorders involves:
• diagnosing and treating the cause or removing the precipitating factors
• controlling seizures with anticonvulsant medications
• recognizing and managing the physical and emotional problems related to the disorder.

Spina bifida

A congenital malformation of the neural tube, spina bifida occurs in approximately 0.2% of all live births. The degree of deformity and resultant neuromuscular involvement determine the extent of functional impairment.

In spina bifida occulta, the vertebral column is incompletely closed and the neural tissue is not displaced. It may be detected incidentally by X-ray or physical examination and may be apparent by a tuft of hair, dimple, or pigmented nevus on the spine. Usually, no treatment is required.

In spina bifida cystica, intraspinal contents protrude through the bony defect. In the meningocele type of spina bifida cystica, spinal fluid and meninges protrude; in the meningomyelocele type, neural tissue and spinal fluid are contained in the cyst.

The defects associated with this disorder usually occur in the lumbosacral area of the spine, but also may occur at other levels. (In the Arnold-Chiari deformity, the meningomyelocele is accompained by hydrocephalus caused by displacement of cranial structures.) Although the exact etiology is unknown, viruses, genetic factors, and such environmental factors as radiation may be involved.

Because children with spina bifida cystica are repeatedly hospitalized for such complications as burns, fractures, decubitus ulcers, urinary tract infections, and shunt failure, you will likely encounter the same children periodically while assigned to the pediatric unit. These children will be well known to the regular nursing staff.

Assessment

Frequently encountered data for spina bifida include the following:
Spina bifida occulta
Although this type usually is asymptomatic, dimpling may be apparent over the sacrococcygeal area of the spine.
Spina bifida cystica
Although this type is readily apparent at birth, full realization of its effects may not occur until the child fails to achieve the devel-

opmental milestones of locomotion and toilet training.

Objective data include:
• various degrees of paresis or paralysis
• sensory deficits
• hydrocephalus (may be evident at birth or develop in the following days with signs of increased intracranial pressure [ICP]; see "Hydrocephalus" in this section)
• possible orthopedic problems, including:
 —kyphosis
 —scoliosis
 —lordosis
 —clubfoot
 —flexion contractures
 —congenital hip dysplasias.

Nursing diagnosis
Altered Thought Processes related to increased ICP
Desired outcome: No evidence of altered thought processes occurs.

Interventions
For a list of associated nursing interventions, see "Hydrocephalus" in this section.

Nursing diagnosis
Potential for Infection related to spinal opening and neural deficits
Desired outcome: The child has no evidence of infection associated with spina bifida.

Interventions
1. Take the following measures to prevent the spread of local infection to other areas (teach these measures to the caregivers and child, if appropriate):
• Carefully cleanse the sac or incision site and apply a sterile dressing.
• Keep the area free of urine or fecal contamination.
• Carefully handle and position the child to prevent traumatizing or rupturing the sac.
• Administer antibiotics, as ordered.
• Monitor the site and report promptly any sign of redness, tears, ulceration, or drainage.
2. Take the following measures to prevent urinary tract infection:
• Provide an acid-ash diet.
• Monitor the child's fluid intake and output.
• Avoid contamination of the urinary meatus with stool.
• Use intermittent catheterization or Credé's method, as ordered, to prevent urine stasis.
• Assist with obtaining specimens for routine urinalysis, urine

culture, and renal function tests, as ordered. (These studies often continue on an outpatient basis.)

• Instruct caregivers on performing Credé's method and on the importance of follow-up laboratory studies.

• Assist with surgical urinary diversion, if ordered.

3. Take the following measures to prevent skin breakdown and infection:

• Provide good skin care and teach the caregivers proper skin care procedures.

• Inspect the child at least two times a day for signs of irritation or trauma, and teach caregivers how to inspect the child.

Nursing diagnosis

Potential for Injury: Trauma related to decreased tactile and temperature sensation

Desired outcome: No evidence of injury occurs.

Interventions

1. Provide anticipatory guidance concerning the following:

• the need for proper-fitting shoes

• keeping the child's crib, playpen, and infant seat well padded

• checking the bathwater temperature before immersing the child's insensitive body parts (The child may be incapable of pain and temperature sensation in the legs and feet because of the neural deficit.)

• keeping the child away from radiators, stoves, and heaters

• avoiding the use of electric blankets

• monitoring the child for chafing and irritation if he is wearing a cast or brace.

2. Take the following measures to prevent and treat fractures, which occur easily because of the child's frail osteoporotic bones:

• Inspect the child after trauma (even minor traumatic events) for redness, swelling, warmth, or deformity because the child will feel no pain.

• Splint any suspected fracture and seek immediate medical attention.

3. Institute the usual interventions for a child admitted for burns, fractures, or other trauma.

Nursing diagnosis

Impaired Physical Mobility related to effects of voluntary motor deficits

Desired outcome: The child has no muscle contractures, atrophy, or injury.

Interventions

1. Assist the child with range-of-motion exercises.

2. Keep the child properly positioned to maintain good body alignment.

3. Teach the caregivers and child (if appropriate) how to perform transfers from a bed to a wheelchair, then back to a bed, using good body mechanics.
4. Take the following measure to prevent falls:
• Keep the crib or bed side rails up and the bed in a low position.
• Secure safety belts if a Stryker frame or Roto Rest bed is used.
• Try to anticipate the child's needs so he won't attempt getting out of bed.
5. Encourage the child and offer support regarding his efforts with occupational and physical therapies. Also, explore with the caregivers and therapeutic team the possibility of the child's using a parapodium walker, creeper, or other device for mobility.

Nursing diagnosis
Impaired Social Interaction related to immobility
Desired outcome: The child interacts freely with others.
Interventions
1. Position the child where he can see others interacting.
2. Read, sing, and talk to the child and encourage the caregivers to do so as well.
3. Allow the child to participate in group activities whenever possible.
4. Help the caregivers with long-term educational planning. (Public Law 94-142 mandates the education of *all* handicapped children.)

Nursing diagnosis
Altered Nutrition: More Than Body Requirements related to immobility
Desired outcome: The child maintains his normal weight for his height.
Interventions
1. Provide a diet high in protein, vitamins, and fluid.
2. Balance the child's nutritional needs with his requirements for bowel and bladder control.
3. Lower the child's total caloric intake if his weight exceeds normal ranges for his height. (*Note:* This is extremely important because excessive weight will interfere with the child's already limited mobility and may become a factor in causing fractures.)

Nursing diagnosis
Altered Bowel Elimination: Bowel Incontinence related to lack of sphincter control
Desired outcome: The child has regular, controlled bowel movements, resulting from successful bowel training.
Interventions
1. Monitor the child's diet to prevent diarrhea or constipation, and provide sufficient bulk for stools.

2. Assess the child's bowel function before training to establish a pattern.

3. To stimulate the bowel reflex, insert a gloved finger in the child's rectum daily, about ½ hour after the predesignated meal (based on the child's established pattern).

4. Insert a glycerin or bisacodyl suppository, and encourage the child to retain it for 15 to 20 minutes.

5. Assist the child to the toilet; teach him to grunt or blow up balloons to increase intraabdominal pressure.

6. Teach the older child to assume responsibility for maintaining his own bowel regimen.

Medical diagnosis

Spina bifida may be diagnosed prenatally based on the following:
• ultrasonography
• increased levels of alpha-fetoprotein in maternal blood.

After birth, a serious defect is obvious; however, the following tests are usually done to determine the extent of neurologic involvement:
• X-ray of the spine
• computed tomography of the skull and spine
• transillumination of the sac to differentiate between meningocele and meningomyelocele involvement
• assessment of the child's reflexes and neurologic responses (tactile and kinesthetic).

Medical treatment

Initial treatment involves closing the sac to prevent infection or trauma and shunting for the existing or ensuing hydrocephalus. Surgery may be performed soon after birth or may be delayed until the child is age 3 months. Simple closure with or without shunting may be sufficient to resolve meningocele without neurologic impairment.

The child with meningomyelocele poses a special challenge. Long-term therapy involves a multidisciplinary approach directed at:
• maintaining the child free of complications
• treating orthopedic problems
• planning for locomotion
• managing excretory functions
• planning the child's education.

☐ Cardiovascular and respiratory systems

Approximately half of all acute childhood illnesses involve respiratory tract diseases. This is because a child's respiratory tract is short, allowing microorganisms fairly direct access into the lungs, and because the immature immune system provides diminished defenses.

Also, because a child's airway has smaller lumen than an

adult's, he is at greater risk for obstruction. Gas exchange also is more readily compromised because the child has fewer alveoli; however, his rapid metabolism demands more oxygen, not less.

Numerous dynamic changes are involved in transforming the fetal heart into one that can function properly in extrauterine life. Sometimes, the heart fails to accomplish all these necessary changes, resulting in circulatory diseases and disorders.

A review of the fetal circulation will help you identify possible cardiovascular deformities; however, a careful history and thorough physical examination are the primary tools of problem identification.

Admission assessment

The cardiovascular and respiratory nursing history usually is tailored to the child's individual needs at the time of admission. If the child is in considerable distress, you'll need to obtain significant information concerning the chief complaint and history of the present illness to provide a data base for initiation of therapy. A complete patient history may be obtained when the child's condition has stabilized.

Patient history. Ask the following questions to obtain a subjective base for your data:
• Chest X-ray: What was the date of the child's most recent X-ray? Why was it done and what were the results?
• Tuberculosis test: What was the date of the last tuberculosis test? What were the results?
• Cough: Does the child have a cough? How often does he cough? Is the cough dry or productive? (If productive, obtain a description of the amount, color, odor, and consistency of the expectorated material.) What time of day does the cough seem to get better or worse? How long do the coughing episodes last?

Inquire specifically about blood in the child's sputum. Does the sputum contain any streaks or clots? Is the bleeding frank? Is the sputum pink and frothy?
• Colds: How often does the child catch cold? What treatment measures are used? (Ask the caregiver to describe a typical cold.)
• Sore throat: Is the child presently complaining about a sore throat, or has he complained of one in the past? How often does this occur? When was the most recent episode? Was it treated? If so, how? What was the response to treatment?
• Voice changes: Has the child had any problems with hoarseness? (When asking about voice changes, allow for normal adolescent changes.)
• Dyspnea: Does the child have any trouble catching his breath? Does he breathe rapidly without physical exertion? If so, under what circumstances? Does he sleep with pillows? How many? Can he sleep without them? Has he ever experienced periods of no breathing?

• Cyanosis: Do the child's lips or fingernails ever turn blue?
• Chest pain: (If pain is present, investigate all the dimensions of symptoms, including region, radiation, precipitating and palliating factors, quality, severity, and chronology.) Does the pain occur on inspiration or expiration? Is it related to activity? Does the child have any tightness of the chest?
• Fatiguability: Is the infant able to suck without tiring? Can the older child keep up with the activities of his peers?
• Smoking: Does anyone in the home smoke? (If the child is older, inquire about his smoking habits.)
• Night sweats, fevers, snoring, exposure to tuberculosis or other infections: Does the child have a history of any of these?
• Allergies: Does the child have any known allergies? Are they seasonal?
• Foreign body aspiration or insertion: Does the child have a history of either?
• Wheezing: Does the child have wheezing or asthmatic attacks? What are the precipitating factors, duration, and usual treatment?
• Congenital anomalies: Are there any known malformations?
• Pain, paresthesias, and anesthesia: Do the child's joints hurt? Are his fingers or toes ever numb or tingling?
• Dizziness or fainting: Does the child ever have spells of dizziness or fainting?
• Heart: Does the child ever have a feeling of pounding or skipped beats? Under what circumstances?
• Medications: Is the child presently taking bronchodilators, cardiotonics, antiarrhythmics, or antihistamines?

Family history. Ask about a family history of the following conditions, which may be considered risk factors:
• congenital heart disease
• hypertension
• tuberculosis
• coronary artery disease
• emphysema
• asthma
• sudden infant death syndrome
• sickle cell anemia
• cystic fibrosis
• leukemia
• obesity
• diabetes.

Physical assessment
This portion of the assessment includes examining the patient to determine his cardiovascular and respiratory status. During the physical examination, be sure to observe and record the following:

Signs of distress. Observe the child for any of the following signs of distress:

- nasal flaring
- circumoral cyanosis
- cyanosis of the nails
- suprasternal, substernal, or intercostal retractions
- tachypnea
- diaphoresis
- paradoxical breathing
- bulging or heaving of the precordium
- distended neck veins
- tachycardia.

Vital signs. Check the child's vital signs. (For specific information on evaluating pediatric blood pressure, see *Taking a child's blood pressure,* page 21.)

Nutritional status and activity level. Weigh the child and measure his height; plot these measurements on a growth grid to determine his percentile. Inquire about the child's typical dietary intake and have the caregivers or child describe the events of a typical day. Be sure to inquire specifically about hobbies, usual activities, and sports.

Skeletal deformities. Observe the child's thorax for any deformities, such as funnel or pigeon chest, kyphosis, or scoliosis.

Allergies. Children with chronic allergies may have characteristic allergic facies. Look for dark circles under the eyes (allergic shiners) and a crease along the lower portion of the nose (allergic salute sign), which is caused by frequent wiping of nasal secretions.

Auscultation, percussion, and palpation. Follow the usual sequence for auscultatation, percussion, and palpation of the child's chest, lymph nodes, and peripheral pulses. Keep in mind the following information:
- Normal breath sounds in smaller children are bronchovesicular because of the proximity of the airways to the chest wall.
- Infants and toddlers often have secretions in the nose because they have not yet learned how to blow them clear. These secretions may result in misleading findings on chest auscultation because of their transmission to the lung fields. Gently aspirate the nares with a rubber ball aspirator or give the child a drink of water, then listen again.
- Breath sounds are best heard with the diaphragm of your stethoscope. However, if you do not have a pediatric stethoscope, the diaphragm may be too large to use on a small child. Instead, you can use the bell of the stethoscope, which will act as a diaphragm if the skin is taut beneath it.
- To facilitate auscultation of a wheeze, apply gentle pressure with your open hand on either the anterior or posterior chest wall during expiration while listening contralaterally.

Asthma

The most common chronic respiratory disorder of childhood, asthma (also known as reactive airway disease) is characterized by smooth-muscle spasms in the bronchi and bronchioles, accompanied by edema and abnormal secretions and resulting in narrowing of the airway.

Considered to have a hereditary predisposition, asthma sometimes is attributed to allergies. Precipitating factors for an attack include upper respiratory infection, stress, and exposure to an allergen. Some children are subject to exercise-induced asthma.

Assessment

Onset of symptoms may be insidious or abrupt. Usually, a child experiencing an asthma attack can be managed in an outpatient setting. Hospitalization is required if the child fails to respond to the usual treatment. If the episode continues despite vigorous treatment, the child is considered to be in status asthmaticus (a severe, prolonged asthmatic attack that does not respond to usual treatment).

Frequently encountered data for asthma include the following:

Subjective
• rapid breathing or inability to catch breath
• fatigue
• feeling of suffocation
• abdominal pain
• occasional vomiting

Objective
• decreased tactile fremitus
• hyperresonant sounds on chest percussion
• tachycardia and tachypnea
• nasal flaring
• wheezing, prolonged expiration, or cough
• anxious expression
• diaphoresis
• restlessness
• use of accessory breathing muscles
• occasional cyanosis.

Nursing diagnosis

Impaired Gas Exchange related to narrowing of the bronchial lumen by spasm, edema, and secretions
Desired outcome: The child has optimal ventilation with no signs of hypoxia.

Interventions

1. Monitor the child for signs and symptoms of persistent or increasing airway narrowing, including:
• diminished breath sounds and increased wheezing
• tachycardia and a drop in blood pressure

• increasing restlessness and anxiety
• vomiting and dehydration
• progressive weakness and fatigue
• cyanosis
• altered level of consciousness
• change in arterial blood gas (ABG) levels indicating acidosis (decreased pH, decreased PO_2, increased PCO_2).
2. Follow doctor's orders to relieve or prevent the above signs and symptoms, including:
• placing the child in high Fowler's position
• administering medications, such as bronchodilators, sympathomimetics, isoproterenol, steroids, antibiotics, or sodium bicarbonate
• providing humidified oxygen
• providing assisted ventilation with a volume respirator, if necessary.
3. After an acute attack, institute the following interventions, if ordered:
• postural drainage
• breathing exercises.

Nursing diagnosis

Anxiety related to severe dyspnea
Desired outcome: The child demonstrates less anxiety, and his dyspnea is relieved or controlled.

Interventions

1. Assess the child's anxiety level by observing for:
• diaphoresis
• restlessness and purposeless movements
• elevation of pulse and respiratory rates
• inability to focus on environmental factors.
2. Provide continuous emotional support with the previously described therapies to provide optimum ventilation. (*Note:* Never leave a dyspneic child unattended.)
3. Administer a sedative, as ordered. (Sedatives may be used judiciously in selected cases.)
4. Provide comfort measures, including rocking, soothing, and touching the child and changing him into dry clothing.

Nursing diagnosis

Knowledge Deficit related to asthmatic disorders and their management
Desired outcome: The caregivers and child (if appropriate) verbalize an understanding of the disease and any environmental or life-style changes necessary to prevent or control asthmatic attacks.

Interventions

1. Provide teaching on the various aspects of the disorder, including:

• its causes. Explore with the family any environmental or life-style factors that may have precipitated the attack. These may include exposure to animals in the home, irritants (such as cigarette smoke), food or other allergens, and intolerance of specific activities, such as vigorous sports or games that require endurance.

• environmental and life-style changes. Explain that the following changes may be necessary to eliminate the risk of precipitating an attack:

—Smoking should be strongly discouraged.

—Pets may need to be eliminated from the home.

—Bedding and pillows must contain no wool or feathers.

—Use of stuffed toys should be discouraged.

—The child's bedroom should be dusted daily with a damp cloth and mop.

—Elimination diets and skin testing may be needed to identify allergens.

—Family counseling may be required to identify and correct stressful relationships and family problems.

—The child may need to switch to sports that require short bursts of energy (such as baseball) rather than endurance events (such as track or basketball). Swimming, almost universally well tolerated by asthmatic children, is highly recommended. (*Note:* The child should be discouraged from adopting a sedentary life-style out of fear of precipitating an attack.)

• medications for long-term management. Make sure the caregivers and child (if appropriate) understand the potential adverse effects of each medication prescribed. Demonstrate the proper use of inhalers; encourage caregivers to monitor inhaler refills with adolescents (overusage is common).

2. Refer the caregivers to the following organizations:

• National Foundation for Asthma, P.O. Box 30061, Tucson, Ariz. 85751

• Asthma Care Association of America, Spring Valley Road, P.O. Box 568, Ossining, N.Y. 10562.

Medical diagnosis

The medical diagnosis for asthma is based on the following:

• the patient history

• clinical findings

• chest X-ray (sometimes required to rule out pneumonia or foreign body aspiration)

• pulmonary function tests

• ABG analysis

• analysis of sputum or nasal secretions (or both) or gastric washing for eosinophils

• skin testing (carried out when the child is symptom-free; involves intradermal injection of small amounts of possible allergens to determine sensitivity; scratch or patch method may be used).

Medical treatment
Treatment goals include:
• administering medications to relieve acute symptoms by promoting smooth-muscle relaxation and decreasing airway secretions and edema, thereby resulting in adequate ventilation
• discovering the cause or precipitating factors and taking steps to eliminate or control them (If elimination of the allergen is impossible, desensitization is a possibility.)
• planning for long-term care. (The child may have to learn to live with asthma but can take measures to prevent or minimize acute episodes.)

Congenital heart defects
Congenital heart defects occur in approximately 8 of every 1,000 live births. Abnormalities of the heart's structure that develop in utero or as the result of hereditary factors, these defects may be classified as cyanotic, acyanotic, or obstructive.

In cyanotic defects, unoxygenated blood is shunted from the right to the left side of the heart, then to all parts of the body. In acyanotic defects, unoxygenated blood is shunted from the left to the right side of the heart. (Children with acyanotic defects show no cyanosis because unoxygenated blood is not transported to the systemic circulation.) In obstructive defects, such structures as valves and vessels are narrowed, resulting in outflow problems and abnormal pressure gradients.

Below is a review of some of the most common defects.

Aortic valvular stenosis. A narrowing of the aortic valve or left ventricular outflow obstruction, aortic valvular stenosis is more common in boys than girls.
Characteristics
• Acyanotic, except in severe defects
• Usually asymptomatic in infants and children
• Severe obstruction results in increased left ventricular pressure to maintain aortic pressure, which in turn may lead to left ventricular hypertrophy
Signs and symptoms
• In infants: atypical systolic murmur and possible intractable congestive heart failure
• Systolic ejection click followed by systolic ejection murmur and a thrill felt at the second right intercostal space or suprasternal notch
• Irritability
• Tachycardia
• Dyspnea and fatigue on exertion

• Angina pectoris
• Syncope
• Pallor
• Narrow pulse pressure
• Weak peripheral pulses
• Possible abdominal pain
• Diaphoresis
• Epistaxis (nosebleed)

Treatment

Surgery may be indicated when myocardial ischemia is present (valvulotomy is the usual surgical procedure); later in life, a prosthetic valve may be necessary.

Atrial septal defect (ASD). Caused by delayed or improper closure of the foramen ovale cordis or atrial septal wall, ASD is characterized by an opening or gap between the left and right atria that allows left-to-right shunting of blood between the chambers.

More common in girls than boys, ASD may be classified as follows:

• ostium secundum—the most common type, located in the fossa ovalis cordis
• sinus venosus—located in the upper atrial septum
• ostium primum—located in the lower atrial septum.

Characteristics

• Acyanotic
• May go unrecognized because of the subtlety of signs and symptoms
• Associated with frequent urinary tract infections
• May interfere with conduction system
• May act as a life-saving safety valve if associated with a severe heart defect, such as transposition of the great vessels
• May cause any of the following:
  —atrial dysrhythmias secondary to right atrial overload
  —pulmonary hypertension if defect is severe
  —complications, including pulmonary thrombosis or embolism, bronchopulmonary infections, and pulmonary artery rupture

Signs and symptoms

• Soft, pulmonic midsystolic murmur heard at the second or third left intercostal space
• In infants: dyspnea on exertion, fatigue, and orthopnea
• In older children with a large defect: left precordial bulge and a frail, delicate appearance

Treatment

ASD may close spontaneously. Treatment usually is supportive until the child is preschool-age or early school-age; direct closure or patch may be done then.

Coarctation of the aorta. More common in boys than girls, this obstructive defect involves constriction of the aorta anywhere on the aortic arch. It is classified as either preductal (if the stricture occurs proximal to the juncture of the ductus arteriosus) or postductal (if the structure occurs distal to the juncture of the ductus arteriosus with the aorta).

Characteristics
• Acyanotic
• Occurrence of symptoms either early in infancy or during young adulthood (usually between ages 20 and 30)
• Possible development of collateral circulation around the defect, which minimizes pressure changes
• In severe defects, possible complications, such as congestive heart failure (CHF), endocarditis, cerebral hemorrhage, aneurysms, or premature arteriosclerosis secondary to hypertension
• Frequently associated with a bicuspid aortic valve

Signs and symptoms
• Elevated blood pressure and bounding pulses proximal to the defect, hypotension, and weak or absent pulses distal to the defect
• Dizziness
• Fainting
• Headache
• Epistaxis
• Cold feet
• Systolic ejection click heard at the base and apex of the heart (associated with systolic or continuous murmur between the scapulae)
• Pulmonary hypertension
• Aneurysm proximal to the defect

Treatment
• Medical treatments include:
  —CHF regimen in infants with preductal coarctation (see *Congestive heart failure,* page 96)
  —balloon angioplasty (A balloon-tipped catheter is advanced through the femoral artery up the aorta to the area of coarctation. The balloon is rapidly inflated and deflated several times, forcing open the area of coarctation. This treatment has been effective in relieving the anomaly.)
  —administration of prostaglandins to infants to maintain a patent ductus arteriosus for shunting of the circulation until surgery is feasible
• Surgery (recommended between ages 4 and 8) involves resection of the aorta with anastomosis or grafting.

Patent ductus arteriosus (PDA). More common in girls than boys, PDA is characterized by a patent duct between the descending aorta and pulmonary artery bifurcation that allows

CONGESTIVE HEART FAILURE

Congestive heart failure (CHF) occurs secondary to other disorders in which the heart cannot meet demands placed upon it. Signs and symptoms include:
• dyspnea at rest
• orthopnea
• paroxysmal nocturnal dyspnea
• costal retractions
• tachypnea
• nostril flaring
• excessive fatiguability (which may affect feeding)
• cough
• diaphoresis
• edema
• enlarged and tender liver
• distended neck veins
• pulsus alternans
• tachycardia with a narrow, thready pulse.

CHF regimen
If your patient has CHF, the doctor may order the following regimen:
• digitalization to slow and strengthen the heartbeat

• inotropic agents to increase or decrease the energy and force of muscle contractions.
• fluid restriction and administration of diuretics to relieve fluid overload
• bed rest to reduce the work load of the heart
• position changes (semi-Fowler's, squatting) to relieve dyspnea
• supplemental oxygen to relieve dyspnea
• emotional support to avoid anxiety and stress, which increase the work load of the heart
• maintenance of normal body temperature (fever increases the work load of the heart)
• meticulous medical asepsis to avoid infection
• small, frequent feedings or gavage to maintain nutrition while avoiding exhaustion
• frequent monitoring of vital signs, potassium levels, hydration status, and weight
• administration of sedatives (may be ordered to reduce demands on the heart when the child is irritable).

shunting of blood from the pulmonary artery to the aorta. Normally, the ductus arteriosus closes shortly after birth.
Characteristics
• Associated with history of prematurity, first-trimester maternal rubella, coxsackievirus infection, or birth at high altitude
• Acyanotic and usually asymptomatic
• May be accompanied by coarctation of the aorta
• May cause pulmonary congestion, especially in premature infants
• May lead to such complications as CHF, ductus arteriosus aneurysm (causing blood to dissect between duct walls), spontaneous aneurysm rupture, and recurrent respiratory infections
Signs and symptoms
• Continuous murmur with characteristic machinelike quality, loudest at the second and third left intercostal spaces; murmur may obscure S_2 heart sounds and may be the only sign of disorder
• Dyspnea on exertion
• Precordial asymmetry; in infants, overactive precordium
• Widened pulse pressure
• Full or bounding pulses
• Pulmonary artery hypertension with right-to-left shunt, and right atrial and ventricular hypertrophy

Treatment
- PDA usually closes spontaneously in the first 3 months of life
- Medical treatments include:
  —administration of indomethacin to induce ductus spasm and closure
  —CHF regimen (see *Congestive heart failure*)
- Surgery (not recommended before age 1) involves ligation and division of the ductus.

Pulmonary stenosis. A narrowing of the pulmonary valve (usually resulting from altered or distorted pulmonary valve cusps or from right ventricular outflow obstruction caused by constriction of the areas immediately above or below the pulmonary valve), pulmonary stenosis is classified as valvular, subvalvular, or supravalvular.

Characteristics
- Usually acyanotic and asymptomatic, except in severe defects
- Associated with a history of maternal rubella
- Causes increased right ventricular pressure to overcome obstruction, which in turn elevates right atrial pressure, leading to increased systemic venous blood pressure
- May result in right ventricular failure
- Associated with low or normal pulmonary artery pressure

Signs and symptoms
- Dyspnea
- Fatigue
- Coldness of the extremities and peripheral cyanosis
- Subjective complaints, such as tiring easily, that increase with age
- Possible precordial pain
- In valvular pulmonary stenosis, systolic ejection murmur associated with a thrill (best heard at the upper left sternal border); in severe defects, murmur may radiate over the precordium and back
- Right ventricular hypertrophy, if right ventricular end-diastolic pressure increases
- Squatting position (assumed by child to relieve respiratory distress)

Treatment
Pulmonary valvulotomy is indicated if right ventricular systolic pressure is markedly elevated; transventricular approach (Boch's procedure) or open heart surgery may be used.

Tetralogy of Fallot. This disorder is actually a combination of four defects: ventricular septal defect (VSD), overriding aorta, pulmonary stenosis, and right ventricular hypertrophy. Tetralogy of Fallot is the most common of the cyanotic congenital cardiac anomalies.

Characteristics
• Shunting of unoxygenated blood through the VSD
• Mixing of oxygenated and unoxygenated blood in the left ventricle, which is pumped out of the aorta, causing cyanosis
• Restricted blood flow to the lungs and increased right ventricular pressure from pulmonary stenosis
• Possible complications, such as iron deficiency anemia, polycythemia, coagulation disorders, paradoxical embolism, cerebral infarction, and abscesses
Signs and symptoms
• Cyanosis
• Loud systolic ejection murmur heard along the left sternal border (may diminish or obscure pulmonic S_2 component)
• Clubbing of fingers and toes
• Dyspnea
• Possible cardiac thrill palpated at the left sternal border
• In newborns: intense cyanosis after PDA closes, severe dyspnea on exertion, syncope, limpness, and occasional convulsions (Untreated defect may prove fatal.)
• Characteristic squatting position (assumed by child to compensate for respiratory distress)
• Respiratory distress and fatigue during feeding
• Growth retardation
Treatment
• Medical treatment includes:
  —administration of oxygen, morphine sulfate, and sodium bicarbonate (to correct acidosis)
  —administration of propranolol prophylactically in children with severe recurrent symptoms
  —administration of prophylactic antibiotics
• Surgery includes:
  —palliative surgery in infancy or early childhood, using procedures designed to shunt blood past the pulmonary stenosis (such as the Blalock-Taussig or Waterston procedure)
  —corrective surgery performed when the pulmonary artery is large enough (usually between ages 4 and 8). Open heart surgery is used to close the VSD and relieve pulmonary stenosis. Antibiotics may be continued indefinitely.

Transposition of the great vessels. Usually associated with VSD, ASD, or PDA, this defect is characterized by transposition of the aorta and pulmonary artery (the aorta leaves the right ventricle; the pulmonary artery leaves the left ventricle). It is more common in boys than girls.
Characteristics
• Associated with history of maternal diabetes
• Causes unoxygenated blood to flow through the right atrium and ventricle and out the aorta to systemic circulation; oxygen-

ated blood flows from the lungs to the left atrium and ventricle and out the pulmonary artery to the lungs
• May cause premature contractions and escape beats
• May be fatal unless VSD, ASD, or PDA exists as a "safety valve" for two independent circulations
Signs and symptoms
• Cyanosis (minimal in infants with a large PDA, or VSD)
• Possible high birth weight
• Signs of CHF, such as dyspnea, within 12 to 24 hours after birth
• Poor sucking reflex
• Systolic murmur if VSD is present
• Hepatomegaly
• Metabolic acidosis from hypoxia (Hypothermia intensifies signs of acidosis.)
Treatment
• Medical treatment (temporary measures until the child is able to undergo surgery) includes:
   —CHF regimen (see *Congestive heart failure,* page 96)
   —administration of prostaglandins to maintain a PDA (if present), or balloon angioplasty to create an ASD
• Surgery involves complex procedures that redirect oxygenated blood to the systemic circulation and deoxygenated blood to the pulmonary circulation. This may be accomplished by transplantation of great vessels to their correct positions or by reversal of atrial functioning.

Truncus arteriosus. Characterized by a single vessel that overrides the ventricles and carries blood for both the pulmonary and systemic circulations, truncus arteriosus results from the failure of the embryonic trunk to separate into the aorta and pulmonary arteries.
Characteristics
• Presence of VSD (always present)
• Possible presence of two to six valve cusps on the common trunk
• Usually fatal within 6 months if untreated
Signs and symptoms
• Cyanosis
• Systolic murmur heard about 1 month after birth
• Fatigue
• Dyspnea
• Failure to thrive
• Parasternal lift
• Possible loud decrescendo diastolic murmur
• Ejection click

• S$_2$ heart sound with only one component because of the presence of a single valve in the common trunk
• Tachypnea
• Crackles
• Recurrent respiratory infections
• Possible wide pulse pressure
• CHF (usually indicating rapid physical decline)
• Possible hepatomegaly
Treatment
Surgery (such as Rastelli's procedure, involving closure of the VSD and excision of the pulmonary arteries from the aorta; pulmonary arteries are attached to the right ventricle) is performed between ages 2 and 3; however, if CHF is severe, surgery must be performed earlier.

Ventricular septal defect (VSD). The most common congenital heart disorder, which occurs more often in premature infants than in full-term infants, VSD is characterized by an abnormal opening in the ventricular septum that allows blood to shunt from the left to the right ventricle.
Characteristics
• Causes oxygenated blood from the left ventricle to mix with unoxygenated blood in the right ventricle (left-to-right shunt). This may serve as a lifesaving measure for a child with more severe heart defects, such as transposition of the great vessels.
• Acyanotic type of defect unless the defect is very large or coupled with another disorder causing right-to-left shunt
• Usually asymptomatic at birth; becomes evident after 2 weeks
• May improve or close spontaneously
• Failure of opening to close within 1 or 2 years after birth may cause pulmonary valve obstruction
• Large opening may eventually cause pulmonary vascular disease and pulmonary artery hypertension; may also result in cardiac complications, such as CHF and bacterial endocarditis
Signs and symptoms
• Overactive precordium, especially after feeding
• Within 6 weeks after birth, harsh systolic murmur (associated with a palpable thrill) heard best in the third and fourth intercostal spaces; child may have no symptoms other than a murmur
• Increased right ventricular and pulmonary artery pressures
• If condition is severe: poor growth and development, labored breathing, and frequent feeding pattern (hungry infant wakes, feeds vigorously, becomes dyspneic, slows and stops feeding, sleeps a short time, wakes, then repeats cycle)
• Recurrent episodes of CHF
Treatment
• May close spontaneously
• Treatment, which depends on the size of the defect and on its

associated symptoms, varies from conservative medical therapy to surgery for simple closure or patch graft.

Nursing diagnosis

Altered Tissue Perfusion related to effects of structural heart defect

Desired outcome: After therapeutic intervention, tissue perfusion is intact to all areas of the body.

Interventions

1. Assess for development or present status of CHF, as indicated by changes in:
• vital signs, including postural blood pressure differences, variations in blood pressure between the upper and lower extremities, and abnormal peripheral pulses
• respiratory distress and hypoxia
• anxiety and restlessness
• hemodynamic monitoring (central venous pressure and pulmonary artery pressure)
• cardiac rhythm
• peripheral edema
• intake and output
• daily weight
• baseline arterial blood gas levels, electrolyte levels, cardiac enzyme studies, and complete blood count
• skin color and turgor
• heart and lung sounds.
2. Take the following measures to maximize tissue perfusion and decrease cardiac workload, thereby relieving dyspnea:
• Provide for quiet and rest (for example, decrease stimuli and carefully schedule all activities and procedures).
• Offer small, frequent feedings of easily digested food.
• Elevate the head of the child's bed unless he has signs of shock.
• Administer medications, as ordered, including inotropics, steroids, antibiotics, vasopressors and vasodilators, diuretics, cardiotonics, and antiarrhythmics.
• Administer oxygen, as prescribed.
• Provide psychological support, including adequate preparation for all procedures.
• Monitor fluid intake.
• Take measures to prevent constipation.
• Keep the child's activity level within recommended limits.
3. Provide preoperative and postoperative care (see Section 4).

Nursing diagnosis

Altered Cardiac Output: Decreased (specify problem) related to effects of structural heart defect

Desired outcome: After therapeutic intervention, cardiac output improves.

Interventions

See the interventions listed for the nursing diagnosis above.

Nursing diagnosis

Potential for Infection: Subacute Bacterial Endocarditis (SBE) related to the abnormal endocardium

Desired outcome: The caregivers identify risks of infection and intervene to prevent their occurrence, and make life-style changes (if necessary) to promote a safe environment for the child.

Interventions

1. Take measures to prevent SBE, and instruct caregivers concerning the need for:
• providing good oral hygiene
• avoiding contact with infected individuals
• performing careful hand washing and other aseptic techniques
• complying with prophylactic antibiotic regimen, when ordered, during times of added risk
• reporting fever or any other signs of illness (because early intervention is vital).

2. During hospitalization of the high-risk child:
• Monitor the child for signs and symptoms of SBE (including fever, malaise, and heart murmur) and any evidence of possible embolic formation (including subonychial hemorrhage and petechiae on the palms, soles, and oral mucous membranes).
• Assist with the following diagnostic tests when SBE is suspected:
   —EKG (may show changes, such as a prolonged PR interval)
   —X-ray (to observe for cardiomegaly)
   —erythrocyte sedimentation rate (elevated during inflammatory process)
   —urinalysis (to check for presence of protein and red blood cells indicative of emboli)
   —complete blood count (to check for anemia and increased white blood cell count caused by infection)
   —blood culture and sensitivity (to identify causative organisms and determine appropriate antibiotic therapy).

3. Provide the following nursing care measures:
• Promote rest, including physical measures and emotional support.
• Administer medications (usually I.V. antibiotics), as ordered. (This includes carefully maintaining a patent I.V. line and observing and reporting any possible adverse reactions.)
• Monitor vital signs and observe for symptoms of congestive heart failure (see *Congestive heart failure,* page 96).

Nursing diagnosis

Dysfunctional Grieving (Parental) related to perceived loss associated with imperfect child

Desired outcome: Parents demonstrate normal progression through the stages of grief, express a desire to understand the problem, participate in the care plan for managing the child's condition, and express realistic optimism and hope.

Interventions

1. Assess all factors involved in the caregivers' grief, including:
• their present stage in the grieving process
• their ability to function at their current anxiety level
• their previous methods for dealing with loss, including their cultural background and support systems.

2. Help the caregivers deal with the perceived loss by:
• encouraging them (without forcing them) to verbalize their feelings, including anger
• being available, showing concern, listening, and allowing them privacy when desired
• encouraging the use of coping strengths (those which have proven effective in previous situations).

3. Provide information on:
• the need for expressing feelings of guilt (if appropriate)
• the normalcy of the grieving process
• the medical condition and plan of care
• referrals for counseling and support.

Medical diagnosis

The medical diagnosis for congenital heart defects is based on:
• the physical assessment and clinical findings
• EKG
• echocardiography
• cardiac catheterization
• arterial blood gas and electrolyte levels
• complete blood count
• cardiac enzyme studies
• chest X-rays
• angiography
• aortography
• scans (such as multiple-gated acquistion scanning)
• pneumocardiography.

Medical treatment

Treatment aims to manage the disorder to provide the child's maximal physical and psychological development. Total correction is ideal but not always possible. When the corrective procedure must be delayed, the medical goal is to maintain the child without complications or deterioration of the condition.

Croup

An acute inflammatory condition of the upper and lower respiratory tracts, croup occurs most commonly in children age 3 months to preschool-age, usually in late fall or early winter. Common causative organisms include influenza, parainfluenza, adenoviruses, and respiratory syncytial virus.

Hospitalization is necessary when fever is high, epiglottitis is suspected, or symptoms of hypoxia occur. In cases of uncomplicated laryngotracheobronchitis (the most common form of croup), the child's symptoms may improve by the time he arrives at the hospital (usually because of exposure to cool, moist air during transport).

Assessment

A child with croup usually has a history of upper respiratory tract infection of several days' duration. Symptoms result from edema and obstruction of the airway.

Frequently encountered data for croup include the following:

Subjective
• fever
• harsh, barking cough
• hoarseness
• restlessness
• worsening of symptoms at night

Objective
• fever
• erythema and edema of the pharynx
• harsh, barking cough
• hoarseness
• diminished breath sounds
• inspiratory stridor
• prolonged expiratory phase
• dyspnea (nostril flaring, tachypnea, and retractions)
• anxiety.

Note: To rule out epiglottitis (sometimes called bacterial croup), observe for and question the caregivers concerning:
• dysphagia
• drooling
• air hunger (Kussmaul's respirations)
• acute onset of symptoms.

If epiglottitis is suspected, do not attempt to examine the child's throat or to make him lie down; this may result in further swelling or spasm, possibly leading to complete airway obstruction.

Nursing diagnosis

Ineffective Gas Exchange related to inflammation and edema of the airway
Desired outcome: The child has no evidence of dyspnea or stridor.

Interventions
1. Carefully observe the child for epiglottitis (see "Epiglottitis" in

this section) and the following signs and symptoms of increasing airway obstruction:
• air hunger
• agitation
• change in level of consciousness
• elevated pulse and respiratory rates
• fever
• cyanosis.
2. Use a croup scoring system or a croup flow sheet, if available.
3. Follow doctor's orders to relieve croup symptoms, including:
• providing bed rest and a calm, quiet environment
• administering antipyretics to control fever
• keeping the child in a humid environment, such as a Croupette or croup tent (the treatment of choice)
• administering racemic epinephrine (2.25% racemic epinephrine in a 1:5 solution with normal saline solution) via intermittent positive-pressure breathing (ordered only if airway obstruction is extreme).
4. Maintain hydration by giving fluids orally (if possible) or I.V., as ordered.
5. Institute orders for treating complete airway obstruction, including maintaining an airway via nasotracheal tube, endotracheal tube, or tracheostomy.

Nursing diagnosis

Knowledge Deficit related to course of croup and home management
Desired outcome: The caregivers describe the cause, signs and symptoms, and home management of croup as well as how to observe for complications.

Interventions

1. Teach the caregivers—especially the primary caregiver—the following information:
• Use of a cool mist vaporizer is preferred to steam because it:
  —produces less hyperemia of mucous membranes
  —will not raise the level of fever
  —is less of a safety hazard (a small child will not be burned if it is accidentally tipped over).
(*Note:* Instruct caregivers to place the child in a steamy bathroom if no vaporizer is available in the house.)
• The child should be encouraged to drink clear fluids.
• Croup is usually self-limited with a good prognosis.
• Inspiratory stridor usually recurs nightly for 2 or 3 nights; other upper respiratory tract symptoms persist for approximately 1 week.
• Recurrences are common, especially when associated with an allergy.

• Medical attention is required if any of the following signs and symptoms of airway obstruction occur:
   —tachypnea
   —cyanosis
   —stridor
   —retractions
   —restlessness
   —increased anxiety.
2. Teach the caregivers how to count respirations and to assess for cyanosis and retractions.

Medical diagnosis

The medical diagnosis for croup is based on the patient history, clinical manifestations, and the child's response to treatment. However, before a positive diagnosis is made, foreign body aspiration, angioneurotic edema, hypocalcemia, and tumor must be ruled out. Frontal and lateral chest and neck X-rays may be ordered.

Medical treatment

Treatment is usually symptomatic and supportive.

Cystic fibrosis

An incurable, inherited autosomal-recessive disease, cystic fibrosis is caused by a generalized dysfunction of the exocrine glands, resulting in abnormally thick secretions that produce obstruction. Such obstruction produces stasis and bacterial growth in the respiratory tract, causing frequent respiratory infections and, eventually, pulmonary fibrosis. In the pancreas, inspissated fluids cause obstruction of digestive enzymes, followed by tissue atrophy and fibrosis of the gland.

Most common in white children, the condition becomes evident early in life. Although many affected children now reach adulthood, the prognosis remains unpredictable.

Assessment

Although signs and symptoms and disease severity vary widely among affected children, frequently encountered data for cystic fibrosis include the following:

Subjective (early in disease)
• dry cough (may be the first symptom)
• diarrhea (usually foul-smelling, bulky, and frothy)
• salty-tasting skin (noticed when kissing the infant)
• recurring respiratory infections
• failure to gain weight

Subjective (later in disease)
• easy fatiguability
• pallor

- cyanosis
- dyspnea
- personality changes and behavioral problems
- easy bruising
- headaches

Objective (early in disease)
- meconium ileus (occurs in 7% to 25% of all newborns with cystic fibrosis), as evidenced by:
  —abdominal distention
  —vomiting
  —dehydration
  —failure to pass stool
- cryptorchidism (not universal, but a common finding)
- symptoms of failure to thrive (usually develop within the first 6 months of life)
- steatorrhea
- prolapsed rectum (usually occurs between ages 6 months and 3 years from weak rectal muscles)

Objective (later in disease)
- height and weight low for age
- nasal polyps
- clubbing of fingers and toes
- delayed sexual maturation
- barrel chest with hyperresonant lungs
- cyanosis
- symptoms of right-sided heart failure and right ventricular hypertrophy
- engorgement of neck veins
- hepatomegaly.

Nursing diagnosis
Ineffective Airway Clearance related to thick mucous secretions and frequent respiratory infections
Desired outcome: The airway remains clear.

Interventions
1. Institute the following medical orders and nursing measures to provide a patent airway and manage respiratory infection:
- Place the child in a mist tent.
- Provide aerosol treatment via an ultrasonic nebulizer.
- Provide postural drainage.
- Provide chest physiotherapy.
- Promote adequate hydration.
- Institute protective isolation measures.
- Administer I.V. antibiotics in the acute phase (usually broad-spectrum antibiotics until culture results are obtained).
- Administer low doses of prophylactic antibiotics orally to children under age 2.

2. Assist with tracheostomy, if ordered.

3. Provide creative teaching on therapies to use at home. Parents can make postural drainage and chest physiotherapy into a game by having the child:
• pretend he is an elephant by bending and twisting his trunk while swinging his arms and legs
• hang upside down on a jungle gym
• tumble and stand on his head.

Nursing diagnosis

Impaired Gas Exchange related to increased airway resistance, uneven ventilation-perfusion ratios, and fibrotic changes in lung tissue

Desired outcome: The child has no signs or symptoms of impaired ventilation and has adequate gas exchange as evidenced by arterial blood gas levels.

Interventions

1. Administer oxygen, as ordered.
2. Monitor arterial blood gas levels.

Nursing diagnosis

Altered Nutrition: Less Than Body Requirements related to malabsorption secondary to failure of pancreatic enzymes to reach duodenum

Desired outcome: The child maintains appropriate height and weight for his age.

Interventions

1. Measure the child's height and weight and plot these measurements on percentile growth charts.
2. Record the number, color, consistency, and size of stools.
3. Monitor hematologic studies for signs of anemia.
4. Institute a dietary regimen that includes:
• a diet high in calories, protein, iron, and sodium and low to moderate in fat.
• water-soluble supplements of vitamins A, D, and E
• vitamin K (if the child has thrombocytopenia)
• dietary supplements, such as Sustacal and Ensure
• pancreatic enzyme replacement
• rest before meals
• teaching for home nutrition.
5. Refer caregivers to the Cystic Fibrosis Foundation, 6000 Executive Boulevard, Suite 309, Rockville, Md. 20852.

Medical diagnosis

The medical diagnosis for cystic fibrosis is based on:
• the family history (disease may not be apparent because cystic fibrosis is autosomal recessive in nature)
• symptoms (listed by the caregivers)

• laboratory findings, including:
  —sweat test (shows sodium chloride level of >60 mEq/liter)
  —pancreatic enzyme levels (decreased in duodenum drainage)
  —stool fat content (elevated)
  —arterial blood gas levels (decreased PO_2 and elevated PCO_2)
• pulmonary function test results (decreased expiratory reserve volume, increased residual volume, decreased vital capacity, and increased functional residual capacity; these results show evidence of disease progression)
• X-ray findings indicating emphysema, atelectasis, or pneumonia (also sinusitis, which may be revealed as the cause of the child's headaches)
• complete blood count (indicating anemia caused by malabsorption).

Medical treatment
The goal of treatment is to help the child and family enjoy as normal a life as possible through respiratory hygiene, adequate nutrition, and psychosocial adaptation. Medications used to treat cystic fibrosis include pancreatic enzymes, antibiotics, and vitamin supplements.

Epiglottitis
Acute epiglottitis, a rapidly progressive infectious condition of the epiglottis and surrounding tissues, is sometimes referred to as bacterial croup. The causative organism is usually *Hemophilus influenzae* type B, although pneumococci or group A streptococci are sometimes responsible.

Children of any age may suffer from epiglottitis; however, incidence is highest among those age 3 to 6. Usually, the condition occurs in winter and is preceded by signs and symptoms of an upper respiratory tract infection. Because death from complete respiratory obstruction is a major threat, epiglottitis represents a medical emergency.

Assessment
Frequently encountered data for epiglottitis include the following:

Subjective
• sore throat
• swallowing difficulty
• breathing difficulty

Objective
• fever
• croupy cough
• drooling
• cyanosis
• retractions

- stridor
- hoarseness
- erythema and edema of the epiglottis
- tripod positioning.

Nursing diagnosis

Ineffective Airway Clearance related to obstruction produced by inflammation and edema of the epiglottis

Desired outcome: A patent airway is maintained or established; the child's respiratory efforts are effective and not labored.

Interventions

1. *Avoid examining the child's throat with a tongue depressor;* this may precipitate laryngeal spasm, resulting in complete airway obstruction.
2. Elevate the child's head.
3. Observe for signs of progressive respiratory distress, including increasing respiratory rate, use of accessory muscles, stridor, cyanosis, and evidence of extreme fear or anxiety.
4. Obtain intubation and tracheostomy equipment, and assist with placement if needed.
5. Assist with identification of the causative organism by obtaining culture specimens (blood or nasopharyngeal), as ordered, after an airway is established.
6. Administer prescribed antibiotics (penicillin-resistant *Hemophilus influenzae* may require chloramphenicol); aggressive I.V. therapy is the usual method.
7. Give the child nothing by mouth, as ordered, to avoid aspiration.

Nursing diagnosis

Impaired Gas Exchange related to hypoxia secondary to respiratory obstruction

Desired outcome: The child demonstrates improved perfusion as evidenced by decreasing cyanosis and alertness.

Interventions

1. Take measures to decrease the child's oxygen demand by:
- enforcing bed rest
- controlling fever
- offering reassurance and support (for both the child and family, because the family may be upsetting the child)
- encouraging parental support and comfort.
2. Monitor for changes in level of consciousness.
3. Provide oxygen, as ordered.
4. Assist with placement and maintenance of an airway, as necessary.

Medical diagnosis

The medical diagnosis for epiglottitis is based on:
- the patient history and observed symptoms

• nontraumatic, direct observation of epiglottal erythema and edema by the doctor using stand-by emergency equipment
• lateral neck X-ray (This usually is avoided unless diagnosis cannot be made otherwise. However, if it is necessary, a doctor and emergency airway equipment must be present. The need for an open airway takes precedence over the need for a definitive diagnosis.)
• blood or nasopharyngeal cultures.

Medical treatment
Goals of treatment include:
• relieving respiratory symptoms and preventing further morbidity or mortality by maintaining or establishing an airway
• reducing inflammation and edema by destroying the responsible organism.

Leukemia
The term leukemia encompasses a number of disorders of blood-forming tissues marked by uncontrolled proliferation of white blood cells (WBCs) and their precursors. Leukemic subtypes are classified according to the predominant leukocyte involved as well as the clinical course.

Acute lymphoblastic leukemia, which carries the best prognosis, accounts for more than 80% of all childhood cases. Acute myelogenous leukemia, with several subtypes, accounts for most of the other leukemias affecting children.

Treatment usually involves medical interventions rather than surgery. However, bone marrow transplant surgery has been used with some success.

Assessment
Frequently encountered data for leukemia include the following:

Subjective (as reported by the child or caregiver)
• fever and malaise
• pallor
• listlessness, weakness, and fatigue
• anorexia and weight loss
• frequent nosebleeds
• easy bruising
• joint pain

Objective
• dyspnea
• tachycardia
• occasional murmur
• petechiae
• elevated WBC count
• anemia
• signs and symptoms of increased intracranial pressure (see

"Hydrocephalus" in this section) caused by invasion of the meninges by WBCs.

Nursing diagnosis

Potential for Infection related to altered blood-forming tissues
Desired outcome: The child has no signs of infection.

Interventions

1. Assess the following:
• environmental hazards for infection
• the child's skin integrity
• signs and symptoms of infection, including fever, chills, and drainage (nasal or pharyngeal or from lesions)
• laboratory culture and sensitivity reports.
2. Implement the following measures to reduce the risk of infection:
• hand washing
• controlling the number of visitors
• using aseptic technique when performing procedures
• having the child turn, cough, and deep-breathe regularly to prevent hypostatic pneumonia
• keeping the child in protective isolation (possibly a filtered environment)
• maintaining adequate hydration
• providing mouth and skin care
• using creative measures to maintain the child's nutritional status
• administering antibiotics, as ordered
• transfusing concentrated leukocytes, when ordered.
3. Take the following steps to promote wellness:
• Teach the child and caregivers how to control the spread of infection.
• Encourage compliance with a long-term prophylactic antibiotic regimen, when prescribed.
• Assist with plans for social activities that do not expose the child to the threat of infection.
• Stress the importance of maintaining good nutritional status as a prevention against infection.

Nursing diagnosis

Activity Intolerance related to fatigue secondary to leukemia
Desired outcome: The child (and caregivers) identifies and participates in essential activities of daily living (as tolerated), demonstrates the ability to alter activities in response to signs and symptoms of infection, and progresses to increased activity levels.

Interventions

1. Assess the following:
• the child's physiologic response to activity by measuring pulse rate and blood pressure

• the child's subjective response to activity, including any fatigue, pain, and weakness
• prioritization of various activities
• the child's emotional and psychological status in regard to intolerance
• the effects of treatment on activity intolerance.
2. Take the following measures to decrease activity intolerance:
• Transfuse red blood cells, if ordered.
• Plan activities to avoid wasting energy.
• Allow for rest periods between activities.
• Provide positive reinforcement for efforts.
3. Instruct the child and caregivers on the signs and symptoms indicating the child's readiness to increase or need to decrease his activity level and on the importance of proper nutrition, hydration, and adequate rest.

Nursing diagnosis

Fluid Volume Deficit related to hemorrhage secondary to decreased platelet production
Desired outcome: The child has no evidence of hemorrhage.

Interventions

1. Take the following measures to evaluate the child's risk of hemorrhage:
• Observe the skin for petechiae and ecchymoses.
• Assess the child's developmental level, temperament, and play activities in terms of potential for injury.
• Monitor vital signs for the following signs and symptoms of hemorrhage: decreased blood pressure, increased pulse rate, and increased respiratory rate.
• Identify risks inherent in treatment, such as injections.
• Evaluate environmental hazards, such as the child's sleeping on a top bunk bed or roughhousing among siblings.
• Monitor platelet count reports.
2. Implement the following measures to promote safety and minimize the threat of hemorrhage:
• Review the child's life-style with regard to potential for injury.
• Teach caregivers how to control bleeding, especially nosebleeds.
• Discuss the need for supervision of play activities.
• Modify care to minimize the potential for injury (for example, provide nonabrasive mouth care and use small-gauge needles for injections).
• Transfuse platelets, as ordered.

Medical diagnosis

The medical diagnosis for leukemia is based on:
• patient history and physical assessment
• evidence of thrombocytopenia

• complete blood count revealing anemia
• peripheral blood smear indicating elevated levels of blastocytes (immature WBCs)
• lumbar puncture to assess for central nervous system infiltration
• liver and kidney function studies to evaluate the child's ability to metabolize chemotherapeutic agents (done before treatment is started)
• bone marrow aspiration or biopsy (shows increased number of immature WBCs).

Medical treatment
Treatment aims to:
• halt the proliferation of WBCs responsible for the leukemia by means of radiation and chemotherapy
• control infection
• treat anemia
• prevent hemorrhage
• provide psychological support for the child and caregivers.

Near-miss SIDS

Sudden infant death syndrome (SIDS), also known as crib death, is a condition in which an apparently healthy infant with a negative history dies suddenly and unexpectedly—usually during sleep. Autopsy reveals no definable cause of death. In near-miss SIDS, the infant is found and revived before the episode has progressed to death.

Infants with this condition are considered at high risk. The following risk factors are associated with SIDS:
• history of one or more apneic episodes
• previous sibling death from SIDS (Risk is five times that of the general population.)
• prematurity
• low birth weight.

Several theories have emerged concerning the etiology of SIDS. According to these theories, some possible causes include:
• chronic hypoxia with periodic apnea
• immaturity of the cardiorespiratory system or abnormal functioning of the autonomic nervous system (or both), resulting in cardiac dysrhythmias
• laryngospasm (possibly from aspiration of gastric contents)
• anaphylaxis
• spinal trauma
• sudden, overwhelming viral infection
• congenital metabolic disorder.

Assessment

Frequently encountered data for near-miss SIDS include the following:

Subjective

The infant is in the following condition when found (before re-suscitation):

• pale, cyanotic, or ashen
• apneic
• limp and seemingly lifeless.

Objective

Depending on the time elapsed between onset of apnea and re-suscitation of the infant, expect wide variations of findings consistent with oxygen deprivation. For example, the resuscitated infant's condition may be within the two extremes mentioned below:

• pink, vigorous, and crying lustily
• obtunded from prolonged hypoxia.

Nursing diagnosis

Fear related to the initial episode of near-miss SIDS
Desired outcome: The caregivers verbalize fears, demonstrate an understanding of the situation, and appear confident and comfortable with apnea monitoring.

Interventions (involving the entire family)

1. Assess the following:

• the family's understanding of the situation and scope of its threat to the family
• appropriateness of the caregiver's affect (feelings) (For example, assess whether the caregiver shows any sign of denial or depression.)
• the resources available within the family and community for coping with the problem and allaying the caregivers' fears.

2. Assist the caregivers in the following ways:

• Spend time listening to the caregivers.
• Provide information on high-risk infants and home monitoring; refer the caregivers to the National SIDS Foundation, 2160 South First Avenue, Maywood, Ill. 60604.
• Teach the caregivers how to use the monitoring equipment, practicing with the model that will be used in the home.
• Encourage the caregivers to express fears and concerns and offer reassurance.
• Teach or provide information on infant resuscitation (see Section 5).
• Practice a simulated scenario of an apneic episode with the caregivers as often as necessary to build confidence in dealing with the situation. (Remind the caregivers that, in most cases, physical stimulation will result in the infant's resuming respirations. However, the caregivers also should know how to perform infant cardiopulmonary resuscitation in case the child fails to respond to stimulation alone.)
• Encourage the caregivers to seek respite occasionally.

• Arrange for follow-up care and access to a 24-hour hotline or emergency resource.

Medical diagnosis
No definitive studies are available for predicting or diagnosing near-miss SIDS. Diagnosis is based on the patient history.

Medical treatment
Treatment includes the use of apnea monitors for high-risk infants. Infants with near-miss SIDS may require supportive therapy and rehabilitation.

Pneumonia, bronchitis, and bronchiolitis
Grouped together because they involve similar nursing challenges, pneumonia, bronchitis, and bronchiolitis are lower respiratory tract diseases usually preceded by an upper respiratory tract infection.

Pneumonia, an inflammation or infection of the lung, occurs in children of all age-groups, most commonly in winter. Sometimes the result of aspiration, this disorder also may result from bacterial or viral (or occasionally fungal) infection.

Bronchitis, an inflammation or infection of the bronchi, usually is not an isolated childhood condition; it commonly occurs as asthmatic bronchitis and tracheobronchitis. Common in early fall among children from infancy to preschool-age, this disorder usually results from viral infection, although it may be precipitated by bacterial or fungal infection or allergy.

Bronchiolitis, an inflammation or infection of the bronchioles (small airways), typically occurs among children under age 2, primarily during the winter. This disorder usually results from viral infection (especially respiratory syncytial virus) but may result from allergy.

Assessment
Frequently encountered data for pneumonia, bronchitis, and bronchiolitis include the following:

Pneumonia
Subjective
• sudden onset of chills and high fever (especially if causative organism is bacterial; onset is more gradual if organism is viral)
• complaints of GI distress
• abdominal pain
• cough
• diaphoresis
Objective
Depending on the causative organism, signs and symptoms vary widely. Below is a list of some common signs and symptoms:
• fever of 103° to 104° F. (39.4° to 40° C.)

- diaphoresis
- tachypnea
- mild to extreme respiratory distress
- retractions
- decreased breath sounds (unilateral or bilateral)
- dullness on percussion over the affected lung tissue.

Bronchitis
Subjective
- skin that feels warm to the touch
- dry, hacking cough for several days followed by a productive cough with chest pain
- worsening of cough at night
Objective
- coarse inspiratory rhonchi that disappear on coughing
- mild fever.

Bronchiolitis
Subjective
- skin that feels warm to the touch
- abrupt onset of wheezing, coughing, and dyspnea
- irritability
- anorexia
Objective
- shallow, rapid respirations
- nasal flaring
- respiratory distress marked by intermittent cyanosis and retractions
- mild fever
- paroxysmal cough
- hyperresonance caused by emphysema
- fine crackles (bilateral)
- decreased breath sounds with prolonged expiration and grunting
- displaced liver border (positioned downward because of lung hyperinflation)
- tachycardia.

Nursing diagnosis
Impaired Gas Exchange related to inflammatory or infectious processes of the airways
Desired outcome: The child has freedom from symptoms of respiratory distress, arterial blood gas levels within normal limits, and no signs or symptoms of hypoxia.

Interventions
1. Continually assess for and report the following signs and symptoms of increasing hypoxia:
- tachypnea
- shallow respirations

• retractions and nasal flaring
• pursed lips
• cyanosis
• decreased breath sounds
• tachycardia
• agitation or decreased level of consciousness
• fatigue and weakness.
2. Institute the following care measures, as ordered:
Pneumonia
• Monitor vital signs.
• Provide a cool mist vaporizer.
• Encourage the child to take fluids.
• Administer antibiotics (usually ordered if causative organism is bacterial, as evidenced by increased white blood cell [WBC] count, or if disorder is associated with a secondary bacterial infection).
• Provide chest physiotherapy.
• Administer antipyretics.
• Avoid administering cough suppressants, except when rest is severely compromised.
• Institute and maintain a patent I.V. for antibiotic administration or rehydration.
• Administer oxygen (using a sliding scale based on arterial blood gas levels).
Bronchitis
• Monitor vital signs frequently.
• Provide supportive, nonspecific treatment.
• Institute postural drainage.
• Institute chest percussion.
• Provide a cool mist vaporizer.
• Administer antibiotics, as ordered, when sputum becomes purulent.
• Administer expectorants.
• Institute incentive spirometry.
Bronchiolitis
• Monitor vital signs frequently.
• Provide cool humidified oxygen.
• Encourage the child to take fluids.
• Institute bed rest with the child in high Fowler's position.
• Institute chest physiotherapy.
• Institute and maintain I.V. therapy for the dehydrated child.
• Provide suction, as needed.
• Assist with endotracheal intubation for severe hypercapnia.
3. Promote rest and take the following steps to conserve the child's energy:
• Provide comfort measures, including frequent position changes.
• Change the child's clothing and bedding frequently to prevent chills. (Mist therapy will cause dampness.)

• Provide psychological and emotional support to relieve apprehension and anxiety.
4. Institute the following special nursing measures:
• Implement respiratory precautions to prevent cross-contamination.
• Provide frequent mouth care because fever and mouth breathing may result in dryness and cracking of the lips and mucous membranes.
• If antibiotics are prescribed, stress the need to finish the full course of medication even though the child appears asymptomatic. (Antibiotics probably will need to be continued after discharge from the hospital.)
• Promote wellness by reviewing risk factors, including discussions on the child's immunization status; encourage inoculation with the pneumococcal vaccine and *Hemophilus influenzae* type B vaccine, especially if the child is enrolled in day care.
• Provide information on the hazards of smoke inhalation, especially with regard to the child's particular disorder; refer caregivers to a local smoker's cessation program. (The development of chronic bronchitis has been directly correlated with smoking in the home.)
• Discuss with the caregivers the family history of allergies, and explore ways to eliminate possible allergens or other irritants from the child's environment.
• Discuss which signs and symptoms of further problems the caregiver should report after the child is discharged from the hospital. Also discuss the importance of follow-up care.

Medical diagnosis
Medical diagnosis is based on the following:
Pneumonia
• markedly elevated WBC count if causative organism is bacterial; slight elevation if organism is viral
• chest X-ray that reveals infiltration and consolidation
• sputum culture (to determine organism)
• tuberculosis test (should always be done)
Bronchitis
• normal or slightly elevated WBC count
• chest X-ray with possible increased bronchovascular markings
Bronchiolitis
• normal WBC count (elevated eosinophil count if disorder is allergic in nature)
• chest X-ray revealing emphysema
• arterial blood gas studies (decreased PO_2, elevated PCO_2).

Medical treatment
Treatment for all three disorders includes:
• discovering the causative organism or agent
• use of specific antimicrobial therapy, when possible

• use of supportive treatment
• preventing severe respiratory compromise or other complications.

Rheumatic fever

A generalized systemic inflammatory disease, rheumatic fever occurs about 1 to 3 weeks after an untreated group A beta-hemolytic streptococcal infection (usually a sore throat). Major manifestations of the disease include carditis, polyarthritis, and chorea. Fatalities (when they occur) usually are the result of carditis with mitral valve (and sometimes aortic valve) stenosis produced by an autoimmune response.

Rheumatic fever, which primarily affects school-age children, has been reported with increased frequency in the United States within recent years. A strong familial influence has been correlated with this disease.

Assessment

Frequently encountered data for rheumatic fever include the following:

Subjective

The following complaints usually are vague and nonspecific:
• fever
• pallor
• listlessness and fatigue
• weakness
• nausea, anorexia, and weight loss
• dyspnea on exertion
• joint pain
• abdominal pain
• spontaneous nosebleeds
• history of colds, sore throat, or impetigo

Objective

• fever
• enlarged, erythematous, hot joints
• erythematous, nonpruritic macular skin rash
• subcutaneous nodules over bony prominences
• carditis accompanied by the following findings:
  —pericardial friction rub
  —accentuated S_3 heart sound
  —signs and symptoms of heart failure (increased heart rate, increased respiratory rate, dyspnea, orthopnea, cyanosis, restlessness, and distended neck veins)
  —systolic murmur (best heard at the apex of the heart)
  —cardiomegaly
  —irregular involuntary movements indicating central nervous system involvement (Sydenham's chorea or St. Vitus' dance).

Nursing diagnosis

Altered Cardiac Output, Decreased: Fatigue related to effects of progressive carditis, which produces valvular dysfunction
Desired outcome: The child's cardiac output remains within normal limits.

Interventions

1. Perform a baseline assessment of the child's vital signs, including monitoring the apical and sleeping pulses, and of general symptoms. Also review laboratory data and provide ongoing assessments; report any untoward changes in signs or symptoms or laboratory values. (Return of the sleeping pulse to normal indicates improvement.)
2. Provide the following care measures, as ordered, to facilitate complete recovery:
• Institute complete bed rest with the head of the bed elevated (if dyspnea occurs).
• Administer aspirin (desired blood level should be 20 to 25 mg/dl) to relieve joint pain.
• Use caution (smooth and unhurried movements) when handling painful joints.
• Administer penicillin, as ordered.
• Provide restful diversion.
• Provide adequate nutrition (increased protein, carbohydrates, and vitamin C) to maintain weight and facilitate growth and tissue repair.
• Administer steroids, if prescribed, and observe for adverse reactions.
• Monitor hydration status, noting daily weight and fluid intake and output.
• Take measures to decrease boredom by providing age-appropriate activities the child can do while confined to bed. (This will aid compliance.)
• Administer oxygen, as ordered.
• Treat congestive heart failure with digitalis, diuretics, inotropic agents, and a reduced-sodium diet, as ordered.
• Institute necessary environmental controls to promote rest.
• Plan comfort measures and hygiene to allow for rest periods.
• Provide emotional support.

Nursing diagnosis

Knowledge Deficit (specify condition and treatment) related to lack of information about disease
Desired outcome: The child and family demonstrate an understanding of the disease process and treatment and implement care to prevent permanent cardiac damage.

Interventions

1. Take the following measures to involve the child and caregivers in plans for home management to ensure compliance and

prevent recurrence or complications:
• Discuss antibiotic treatment, which usually is continued on a long-term basis.
• Clarify the specifics of the activities permitted.
• Teach comfort and safety measures.
• Plan for home tutoring to maintain school status.
• Provide instruction on signs and symptoms of disease recurrence or complications.
• Encourage follow-up visits.

Medical diagnosis

The medical diagnosis for rheumatic fever is based on:
• clinical findings
• elevated erythrocyte sedimentation rate
• elevated antistreptolysin O titers or other antibody tests
• elevated white blood cell count
• indications of mild anemia
• positive throat culture for beta-hemolytic streptococcal infection
• positive C-reactive protein level
• EKG showing a prolonged PR interval suggestive of carditis.

Medical treatment

Treatment includes the following:
• administration of antibiotics to eliminate beta-hemolytic streptococcal infection
• relief of pain and discomfort
• prevention of recurrences of disease
• prevention of residual cardiac disease.

Sickle cell anemia

A severe, chronic hereditary hemolytic anemia, sickle cell anemia is characterized by crescent- or sickle-shaped fragile red blood cells (RBCs) with impaired ability to transport oxygen. Rarely affecting white children, this disorder affects 1 of every 500 black children born in the United States.

Sickling of cells results in vaso-occlusion, infarction, and necrosis of body organs and joints. Children experiencing episodes of sickle cell crisis present with various symptoms; episodes vary in severity and frequency of occurrence. The most common crisis, resulting in admission of the child to the pediatric unit, involves a painful episode of vaso-occlusion or severe anemia. Severe anemic crises occur because of increased destruction and decreased production of RBCs as well as pooling of blood in the spleen.

Sickle cell anemia usually is not discovered before age 6 months unless the infant is screened beforehand based on a family history of the disorder. Hemoglobin screening may be done prenatally through amniocentesis or at or after birth through cord blood sampling. About half of all infants who test positive are symptomatic by age 1.

A child with sickle cell trait (HbSA) is a carrier of the disorder and does not have sickle cell anemia (HbSS). Although the HbSA child may never present with symptoms, under special hypoxic conditions (such as conditions produced by infection, extreme physical exertion, anemia, high altitude, or anesthesia) symptoms associated with sickle cell anemia may occur.

Assessment
Frequently encountered data for sickle cell anemia include the following:

Subjective
• abdominal pain
• headache and dizziness
• fever
• priapism
• vomiting
• weakness and fatigue
• pallor
• anorexia
• extremity and joint pain
• recent history of upper respiratory tract infection or GI infection

Objective
• tachycardia
• cardiomegaly
• systolic or diastolic murmur
• dyspnea
• joint edema
• symmetrically swollen hands and feet
• hepatomegaly
• splenomegaly
• hematuria
• jaundice or pallor.

Nursing diagnosis
Altered Tissue Perfusion related to hypoxia secondary to anemia, ischemia, or infarction of the involved tissue
Desired outcome: The child has improved tissue perfusion and no evidence of necrosis; he shows pain relief and is restored to his pre-episodic level of functioning.

Interventions
1. Observe, record, and report the following signs and symptoms indicative of ischemia, shock, cerebrovascular accident, or increasing anemia:
• deepening jaundice
• decreased blood pressure

• increased pulse and respiratory rates
• severe pain
• altered mental status
• fever
• mottling, coolness, or cyanosis of the extremities with poor capillary refill and diminished pulses
• respiratory distress
• oliguria or hematuria
• deterioration in laboratory values.
Note: Avoid palpating the child's abdomen; sequestered RBCs may precipitate splenic rupture.
2. Implement the following nursing and medical measures to maximize tissue perfusion and to provide support and protection:
• Institute bed rest to reduce oxygen utilization.
• Administer oxygen, as prescribed, on a short-term basis to break the hypoxia-metabolic acidosis-sickling cycle (in which hypoxia causes metabolic acidosis, which causes sickling; this cycle is then repeated). Long-term oxygen therapy will depress erythropoiesis.
• Provide hydration, either orally or I.V., to promote hemodilution and maintain electrolyte balance.
• Position the child for comfort and maximum blood flow.
• Administer pain medications, as ordered.
• Avoid clothing the child in restrictive garments.
• Avoid exposing the child to chills.
• Encourage supervised exercises within limited recommendations to promote circulation.
• Administer antibiotics, as ordered.
• Monitor blood transfusions for replacement or exchange, as ordered.

Nursing diagnosis
Potential for Infection: Osteomyelitis related to chronic hypoxia of bone
Desired outcome: The child or caregiver verbalizes an understanding of the factors that increase the risk of vaso-occlusive episodes resulting in hypoxia and takes precautions to avoid such episodes and possible bone disease. (Early recognition and treatment of osteomyelitis will result in bone healing, reduced pain, and absence of deformity.)

Interventions
1. Teach the child and caregivers about sickle cell anemia and how to prevent crises.
2. Assess for early signs by taking the following measures:
• Survey the child's skin and report any lesions.
• Observe and report the following signs of inflammation over

bone: pain, edema, and erythema.
• Assess for fever.
3. Monitor the child for the following signs of septicemia: malaise, chills, vomiting, and fever.
4. Expedite any diagnostic tests, including X-rays, blood culture, and complete blood count, as ordered.
5. Administer antibiotic, analgesic, or antibacterial medications, as ordered.
6. Maintain the child's traction, splints, and positions, as ordered.
7. Assist with preoperative and postoperative care if surgical drainage becomes necessary.

Nursing diagnosis
Knowledge Deficit related to lack of information or misinterpretation of medical instructions
Desired outcome: The child and family verbalize understanding of the information presented, identify exacerbating factors, and demonstrate appropriate behaviors to prevent crises.

Interventions
1. Assess the child's and family's knowledge as well as their interest level and ability to learn. Also identify which caregiver has the best potential for learning.
2. Provide the following information concerning the prevention of crises:
• Knowing the signs and symptoms of infection, illness, and crisis is important; providing early intervention is essential.
• The child should avoid stress because it produces vasoconstriction. (*Note:* Enuresis, common among children with sickle cell anemia, is caused by the intake of increased amounts of fluid and the decreased ability of the kidneys to concentrate urine; this can be a source of great stress to children if caregivers are not understanding of the situation.)
• Overprotection of the child with sickle cell anemia can be a source of stress to the child.
• Hydration must be promoted. (Discuss signs and symptoms of dehydration.)
• The child should be protected against infection by avoiding exposure to infection, receiving prompt attention to breaks in the skin, maintaining an immunization schedule, and receiving proper nutrition.
• Moderate physical activity is permitted (usually with the child participating within his tolerance limits).
• Medical follow-up must continue on a regular basis.
3. Suggest the following to the caregivers, as appropriate:
• genetic counseling
• psychological or family counseling if the family demonstrates evidence of guilt or disintegration
• support or information resources.

Medical diagnosis

The medical diagnosis for sickle cell anemia is based on:
• complete blood count (to detect infection or anemia)
• blood smear (may reveal sickled cells)
• urinalysis (checking for proteinuria, hematuria, and decreased specific gravity)
• X-ray (to check for hyperplasia, congestion of bone marrow, and such bone changes as "hair on end" appearance of the skull)
• tests for sickle hemoglobin, including:
   —Sickledex (solubility test; screening is nonspecific for trait or disease)
   —sickling test (sickle cell preparation; screening is nonspecific for trait or disease)
   —hemoglobin electrophoresis (in which high-voltage electricity causes hemoglobin variants to separate; test is done after a positive result from one of the screening tests. Trait is distinguished from anemia as follows: child with trait has approximately 35% hemoglobin S; child with disease has about 80% to 95% hemoglobin S.)
   —enzyme assay (performed through amniocentesis on fetal DNA; detects sickle cell anemia as early as second trimester).

Medical treatment

Treatment may include the following:
• crisis prevention (by maintaining hemodilution and oxygenation with the participation of the child and caregivers)
• management of crisis episodes to prevent irreversible changes
• bone marrow transplant (has resulted in some success with selected cases; however, numerous problems are inherent with this approach)
• hyperbaric oxygen therapy (used successfully in research on individuals with sickle cell retinopathy; however, its effectiveness has not been established for general therapy).

☐ Gastrointestinal and endocrine systems

Diseases and disorders of the gastrointestinal (GI) tract are among the most common illnesses affecting children. Alterations in nutrition and elimination, resulting from impaired structure or function of digestive metabolic processes, threaten both the immediate and long-term health status of the child.

The primary function of the GI tract—providing the body with a steady supply of nutrients, water, and electrolytes—may be impeded by structural and obstructive defects, inflammatory and malabsorptive conditions, or impaired digestive status. The life-threatening implications of fluid and electrolyte imbalance are in themselves a common reason for hospitalization of children.

Altered cellular function resulting from digestive or metabolic disturbances may have profound implications on a child's developmental progress. Diabetes mellitus is the most common endocrine disorder during childhood.

Admission assessment

Ask the caregivers or child (as appropriate) the following questions to establish a subjective data base for assessing the GI and endocrine systems:

Patient history. Ask the caregivers about the following:
• Appetite: Has the child experienced any recent changes in appetite? Any weight loss or gain? If so, how much and how fast? What is the child's usual diet? Has the child ever exhibited pica (the desire to eat nonfood substances)?
• Nausea and vomiting: What were the circumstances and amount? (Ask for a description of the vomitus.)
• Indigestion: Has the child ever had heartburn, belching episodes, distention, or gas pains? Does he have any food intolerances? Does he use any medication?
• Stools: What is the usual frequency, color, and consistency? Does he ever experience bleeding, diarrhea, constipation, or flatus? Has he been infected with parasites? Is the child toilet-trained? Does toilet training have any relationship to onset of symptoms? Does the child use any medication?
• Abdominal pain: Where is the pain located? Does it radiate to other areas? What is the quality of the pain (such as cramping or stabbing)? What is the relationship of the pain's timing to meals or other activities? Have any treatments been tried?
• Jaundice: Has the child ever had jaundice? If so, how long did it persist?
• Tumors or masses: Has the child or caregiver noted any "lumps in the tummy"?
• Dysphagia: Does the child have difficulty swallowing?
• Fever: Has the child ever had a fever? What was the temperature and how long did it last? Was any treatment used?
• Heat or cold intolerances: Does the child ever show signs of intolerance to heat or cold?
• Energy level: Is the child lethargic? Overactive? Is he able to keep up with peers?
• Polyuria, polydipsia, polyphagia: Has the child ever had problems with these?
• Growth pattern: How does the child compare with siblings? Are family members generally large, average, or small? Has the child undergone any recent spurts or declines?
• Sexual development: Does the child have any axillary or pubic hair? Has the female child reached menarche or thelarche (breast budding)? At what age?

Family history. Ask the caregivers about a family history of:
• diabetes
• growth disorders
• ulcerative disorders
• tumors
• hernias
• digestive diseases
• cystic fibrosis
• phenylketonuria (PKU) or other metabolic disorders
• congenital anomalies.

School-related factors. Inquire about the child's academic progress and social activity.

Physical assessment

Because nutrition and hormonal control greatly affect a child's growth and development, serial growth charts are extremely important when assessing the GI and endocrine systems. Keep in mind that unsatisfactory nutritional status is reflected in inappropriate development. Using the Denver Developmental Screening Test (DDST) will provide information useful to your development of a data base.

To assess the child's abdomen, you'll need a stethoscope, a ruler, and a marking pencil. If a rectal examination is indicated, you'll also need gloves and a lubricant; however, this type of examination is not routine for the child. Because the child's relaxation is key to a satisfactory abdominal assessment, you may find it easier to allow the child to remain on the caregiver's lap after first assessing the abdominal contour while the child is standing. Be sure to warm your hands before beginning the examination.

While performing the physical assessment, use the following examination techniques:

Inspection. Note the child's skin color and any signs of scarring. Also note the venous pattern. Check for signs of hernia (umbilical or inguinal) and visible peristalsis. Also check for evidence of diastases of the abdominal muscles. Note the presence of pubic hair.

Auscultation. Listen for the presence, timing, and quality of bowel sounds in all four quadrants. Also listen for bruits, murmurs, or a venous hum.

Percussion. Use percussion to check for gastric tympany, locate the liver border, and detect splenic dullness (may extend 1 to 2 cm below the costal margin in an infant or young child).

Palpation. Begin with superficial palpation, followed by deep palpation to assess abdominal rigidity or guarding. Palpate for femoral or inguinal hernia. Also palpate for skin texture and turgor. Note any abdominal tenderness, describing its location, depth, and rebound quality.

Pulsations. For aortic pulsations, note the size and location of the pulse. For femoral pulsations, note symmetry and amplitude.

Inspection and palpation of masses. Describe the location, size, consistency, mobility, and contour of any palpable masses. Note their relationship to abdominal organs as well as any associated symptoms, such as tenderness.

Appendicitis

The most common reason for abdominal surgery in children, appendicitis involves inflammation of the vermiform appendix, which is located in the right lower quadrant of the abdomen at the end of the cecum. In appendicitis, the inflamed appendix becomes obstructed, causing increasing pressure, ulceration of the abdominal lining, and bacterial invasion. Eventually, tissue necrosis leads to rupture. A child's immature abdominal structures allow peritonitis to spread readily to accessory GI and reproductive organs.

Rarely occurring in children under age 2, appendicitis often is difficult to diagnose in small children. Frequently, sufficient time elapses before diagnosis to allow the appendix to become perforated. Also, because the child may by unable to describe symptomatic changes, caregivers of young children may delay seeking treatment. Health care providers must be alert to significant symptoms.

Assessment

Frequently encountered data for appendicitis and peritonitis include the following:

Appendicitis

Subjective
• abdominal pain (at first generalized or periumbilical, then descending to the right lower quadrant)
Objective
• fever
• rebound tenderness and abdominal rigidity
• decreased or absent bowel sounds
• vomiting
• diarrhea or constipation
• irritability
• side lying with knees flexed, hesitancy to move (sometimes displayed by a nonverbal child)

Peritonitis

• increased pain (after a period of relief), followed by abdominal rigidity and distention
• rapid, shallow breathing
• increased fever.

Nursing diagnosis

Altered Comfort related to abdominal pain, nausea, and vomiting secondary to preoperative inflammatory process and postoperative recovery

Desired outcome: The child has diminished pain as evidenced by verbalization as well as by relaxation of expression and body rigidity; the child also has relief of nausea and vomiting as evidenced by verbalization and absence of vomiting.

Interventions

1. Assist the child to a comfortable position, such as a side-lying position with the right knee flexed. (This position reduces tension of the abdominal musculature over McBurney's point.)
2. Monitor for effects of analgesics.
3. Change the child's position slowly.
4. Maintain food and fluid restrictions, as ordered. (The child will not be able to have anything by mouth preoperatively.)
5. Provide frequent oral care.
6. Monitor for effects of antiemetics.

Nursing diagnosis

Potential for Infection related to development of peritonitis or abscess formation secondary to fecal contamination of abdominal cavity

Desired outcome: Peritonitis or abscess resolves as evidenced by the child's normal temperature, absence of abdominal pain or cramping, normal bowel sounds, and normal white blood cell (WBC) count.

Interventions

1. Monitor for the following signs and symptoms of peritonitis:
• fever
• increased and more constant abdominal pain
• increased pulse and respiratory rates
• decreased blood pressure
• increased WBC count.
2. Use appropriate measures to control existing infection or to limit its extension.
3. Take the following measures if drains are in place postoperatively:
• Maintain the patency of drains.
• To prevent inadvertent drain removal, keep the child from pulling on tubing.
• Keep the dressing dry and clean.
• Empty the wound drainage bag.
4. Place the child in Fowler's or semi-Fowler's position.
5. Prevent other complications by having the child turn, deep-breathe, and cough every 2 hours, and by having him walk as ordered.

Medical diagnosis

The medical diagnosis for appendicitis is based on:
• the patient history and physical examination findings
• elevated WBC count
• abdominal X-ray.

Medical treatment

Treatment for appendicitis includes surgical removal of the appendix.

Treatment for peritonitis includes:
• measures to manage shock, dehydration, and infection (preoperatively and postoperatively)
• administration of I.V. fluids and systemic antibiotics
• nasogastric suction (to keep the GI tract at rest).

Cleft lip and palate

The most common congenital facial malformation, cleft lip is caused by defective development of the anterior maxilla or the palate. Cleft lip may be unilateral or bilateral and can occur with or without cleft palate. A cleft palate may involve only the uvula or may extend through the soft and hard palates. Although severity and extent varies, the clefting creates feeding problems and also may cause speech defects.

Assessment

The degree of cleft lip is identified visually and may include nasal distortion. Cleft palate alone may be recognized by the child's difficulty in feeding and may be identified by the examiner's fingers.

Nursing diagnosis

Altered Nutrition: Less Than Body Requirements related to inability to develop suction when feeding or difficulty in swallowing
Desired outcome: The infant receives adequate nutrition in as normal a feeding situation as possible.

Interventions

1. Feed the child in an upright position.
2. Use special nipples or feeding devices.
3. When a feeding tube (gastric intubation) is required, meet the child's sucking needs with a pacifier.
4. Allow the child to burp frequently.

Nursing diagnosis

Impaired Skin Integrity related to effects of surgical incision
Desired outcome: The child has uncomplicated wound healing as evidenced by minimal disability and disfigurement.

Interventions

1. For cleft lip, position the child on his back or side; for cleft palate, position the child on his abdomen.

2. Maintain a lip protective device.

3. Restrain the child's arms to prevent access to the operative site.

4. Cleanse the suture line gently after feeding and as indicated; keep the area dry.

5. Provide gentle aspiration of mouth and nasopharyngeal secretions.

Nursing diagnosis

Anxiety (Caregivers) related to child's appearance and difficulty in feeding

Desired outcome: The caregivers verbalize decreased anxiety about meeting the infant's needs.

Interventions

1. Convey an accepting attitude.

2. Encourage the caregivers to express their feelings.

3. Demonstrate and teach feeding, wound protection, healing, and suctioning techniques.

4. Demonstrate cuddling and tactile stimulation.

5. Involve the caregivers in the infant's care; remain at the crib side to provide support.

Medical diagnosis

The medical diagnosis for cleft lip and palate is based on inspection and palpation and radiographic examinations.

Medical treatment

Treatment goals include:

• closure of the cleft (Optimum time for surgical correction of cleft lip is by age 1 month; for correction of cleft palate, by age 6 months.)

• prevention of complications, such as malnutrition and aspiration

• facilitation of growth and development.

Treatment will need to be continued over a long period of time. Residual speech defects and altered facial appearance may be unavoidable.

Diabetes mellitus

The most common childhood disorder of the endocrine system, insulin-dependent diabetes mellitus (IDDM), also known as Type I diabetes, is a chronic disease of insulin deficiency or resistance.

Essential for cellular metabolism of carbohydrates, fat, and protein, insulin prevents the mobilization of fat from fat cells and allows storage of glucose as glycogen in liver and muscle cells. Because of the unavailability of glucose for fuel, the body relies on fat or protein as a fuel source, resulting in a state of catabolism and ketosis. Elevated blood glucose levels, resulting from decreased glucose utilization, leads to the development of extracellular and intracellular dehydration.

If poorly controlled, IDDM causes damage to tissues of the vascular and nervous systems as evidenced by retinopathy, nephropathy, and neuropathy.

Assessment

Frequently encountered data for IDDM include the following:

Subjective

• behavioral changes (for example, the child may be grouchy or "not himself")
• excessive tiredness
• complaints of abdominal discomfort (often mimicking gastroenteritis, appendicitis, or flu)

Objective

• family history of diabetes
• increased hunger, thirst, and urination
• weight loss from dehydration or malnutrition
• dry skin, blurred vision, and poor healing of sores.

Nursing diagnosis

Fluid Volume Deficit related to excessive loss from diarrhea, vomiting, and osmotic diuresis

Desired outcome: The child maintains fluid balance as evidenced by normal skin turgor and moist mucous membranes, balanced intake and output, usual mental status and neuromuscular function, and vital signs within the normal range.

Interventions

1. Monitor the child's skin turgor, intake and output, vital signs, urine specific gravity, mental status, neuromuscular status, and serum electrolyte levels.
2. Reduce environmental stimuli, change the child's position slowly, and explain and assist with dietary restrictions.
3. Administer medications, such as insulin, fluids, electrolytes, antiemetics, antidiarrheals, and alkalizing agents, as ordered, and monitor their effects.
4. Test the glucose level in urine or blood (or both).
5. Monitor for the following signs of ketoacidosis:
• fruity breath odor
• warm, flushed, and dry skin
• lethargy or stupor
• changes in blood gas levels.
6. Maintain bed rest during the child's ketoacidotic state.
7. Implement active or passive leg exercise every 2 hours.
8. Monitor the child for the following signs of hypoglycemia:
• cool, clammy skin
• mood swing (jitteriness and irritability)
• evidence of nightmares
• absent squint reflex from light during sleep.

If signs and symptoms of hypoglycemia occur, administer a rapid-acting carbohydrate, such as orange juice, apple juice, or a soft drink. If the child is unresponsive and cannot swallow, follow your usual hospital protocol (for example, administer a 50% glucose solution I.V.).

9. Provide emotional support to the child and caregivers.

10. Anticipate the need for alternate forms of nutritional intake and changes in insulin requirements in response to illness, diagnostic tests, or surgery.

11. Help the child return to his usual activity level as soon as possible.

Nursing diagnosis

Knowledge Deficit (Child or Caregivers): Noncompliance with Long-term Care related to lack of understanding and anxiety about care regimen

Desired outcome: The child or caregivers comply with the regimen and verbalize an understanding of and less anxiety about long-term care.

Interventions

1. Explain diabetes and its treatment in terms the child and caregivers can understand.

2. Involve the child and caregivers in establishing a care schedule that encompasses maintaining an adequate diet, balancing activity and rest, maintaining skin integrity, monitoring glucose levels, and administering insulin.

3. Teach the child and caregivers how to administer insulin and monitor blood glucose levels. (Teach the child as early as possible, preferably by age 3 to 4.)

4. Provide information concerning community resources and support groups.

5. Establish a therapeutic relationship with the child and caregivers. Be available to listen, talk, and provide comfort and support.

Medical diagnosis

The medical diagnosis for IDDM is based on:
• clinical signs and symptoms
• fasting blood sugar (FBS) levels; however, the FBS levels may not detect early or asymptomatic diabetes
• glucose tolerance testing (4- or 6-hour testing)
• serum electrolyte levels, blood gas levels, and EKG to monitor acute problems
• hemoglobin A_{1c} levels.

Medical treatment

Treatment aims to:
• balance blood glucose levels through the integration of insulin, diet, and activity

• maintain as normal a physiologic state as possible (while avoiding a pattern of rigidity that may be uncomfortable to the child and family) and 24-hour insulin coverage based on the child's individualized needs.

Medications administered during episodes of illness or mismanagement include regular insulin, plasma expanders, and fluids and electrolytes. Maintenance insulin includes a combination of intermediate-acting insulin (given once a day) with regular insulin (given at regular intervals based on a sliding scale in response to blood glucose levels). (See *Comparing insulins.*)

Treatment for diabetic ketoacidosis, a life-threatening complication, includes:

• reversing the condition by administering insulin (regular insulin may be preferable), fluids, and electrolytes

• providing nursing management during illness, surgery, or other stressful situations

• adjusting insulin and dietary intake to compensate for changes in blood glucose levels.

COMPARING INSULINS

Insulin	Onset of action	Peak effect	Duration of action
Rapid or short-acting regular (Actrapid, Humulin R, Regular Iletin)*	½ to 1 hour	2 to 3 hours	5 to 7 hours
Rapid zinc (Semilente, Semitard)	½ to 1 hour	4 to 7 hours	12 to 16 hours
Intermediate-acting NPH (Humulin N, NPH Iletin)	1 to 2 hours	8 to 12 hours	18 to 28 hours
Intermediate zinc (Humulin L, Lentard, Lente, Monotard)	1 to 2 hours	8 to 12 hours	18 to 28 hours
Long-acting protamine zinc insulin (PZI)	4 to 8 hours	14 to 20 hours	36 hours
Extended zinc (Ultralente, Ultratard)	4 to 8 hours	16 to 18 hours	36 hours

*Only regular insulin may be given I.V. If given I.V., onset is 10 to 30 minutes; peak effect, 15 to 30 minutes; and duration of action, 30 to 60 minutes.

Gastroenteritis, acute

A nonspecific admission diagnosis, gastroenteritis is character-ized by nausea, vomiting, and diarrhea. The ensuing dehydration and electrolyte imbalance that develops from these symptoms may be life-threatening to the infant or young child and may ne-cessitate hospitalization.

Identification of the underlying cause is essential to treatment. The infant or child hospitalized with nonspecific diarrhea must be isolated to prevent spreading of a possible pathogen to other patients and personnel.

Causes of acute diarrhea, with or without vomiting, include en-teropathogens (such as *Escherichia coli, Salmonella,* or *Shigella*), ingestion of toxins, dietary indiscretions, and other infectious or communicable diseases.

Assessment

Frequently encountered data for acute gastroenteritis include the following:

Subjective
• abdominal cramps
• headache
• nausea (in an older child)

Objective
• frequent, watery stools (usually greenish, possibly containing mucus)
• hyperactive bowel sounds
• vomiting
• signs and symptoms of dehydration, including:
—decreased urine output
—electrolyte imbalance
—depressed fontanelles
—sunken eyeballs
—loss of tissue turgor
—dry mucous membranes
—weight loss
• signs of systemic infection.

Nursing diagnosis

Altered Bowel Elimination: Diarrhea related to hyperactive peri-stalsis or bowel inflammation
Desired outcome: Bowel elimination returns to normal as evi-denced by improved consistency and decreased frequency of stools.

Interventions
1. Maintain food and fluid restrictions, as ordered.
2. Apply a urine collection bag to the infant or incontinent young child.
3. Estimate output by weighing soiled or wet diapers, then sub-

tracting the weight of a dry diaper from the weight of the used diaper. (*Note:* 1 gram of weight equals 1 milliliter of liquid.)
4. Monitor bowel sounds.
5. Encourage rest and sleep, and limit disturbances for assessment and care.
6. Cleanse the perianal area immediately after defecation to prevent skin excoriation.
7. Instruct caregivers in the safe handling and proper disposal of the child's excreta and of soiled diapers, tissues, and other waste.
8. Institute special mouth care.

Nursing diagnosis
Fluid Volume Deficit related to excessive loss through diarrhea or vomiting
Desired outcome: The child has normal skin turgor, moist mucous membranes, balanced intake and output, and stable body weight.

Interventions
1. Monitor for signs and symptoms of fluid and electrolyte imbalance (see "Fluid and Electrolyte Imbalance" in the Appendices).
2. Take and record the child's daily weight.
3. Monitor urine specific gravity and volume.
4. Monitor the intake of parenteral fluids and electrolytes.
5. Assess the child's reaction to resuming oral intake (usually glucose or electrolyte solution), and discontinue feedings if diarrhea persists or returns.
6. Assess the child's reaction to the addition of milk to the diet (should be progressed cautiously) in case of altered lactose tolerance.
7. Reassure caregivers and encourage them to provide comfort measures when the child's activity is restricted.
8. Administer mouth care after episodes of vomiting.

Medical diagnosis
The medical diagnosis for acute gastroenteritis is based on:
• identification of the cause of vomiting or diarrhea (based on history and physical examination)
• cultures and laboratory analysis of stool specimens for ova and parasites.

Medical treatment
Treatment includes:
• rehydration to rapidly restore circulating fluid volume (severe diarrhea may be fatal to children)
• assessment of electrolyte imbalance and administration of replacements to restore normal levels
• treating the underlying cause with antimicrobials, dietary restrictions, or sedation, as appropriate.

Hernia

Hernia refers to the protrusion of abdominal contents through openings in the midline or lower abdominal wall. Inguinal hernia, the most common type of hernia in infancy, is present at birth and usually becomes apparent at age 2 to 3 months. Most common among boys, inguinal hernia usually is repaired in otherwise healthy infants immediately after diagnosis to avoid possible complications of incarceration and strangulation.

In umbilical hernia, surgery is indicated only after age 2 (girls) or age 4 (boys) when the hernia does not resolve spontaneously. The umbilical ring defect, which is responsible for this type of hernia, varies in size.

Other types of hernias in children include omphalocele and gastroschisis. Omphalocele, a birth defect at the base of the umbilicus, is characterized by a protrusion of the abdominal viscera, which is covered by a thin abdominal membrane. Gastroschisis refers to herniation of the viscera through the abdominal wall (the viscera is not enclosed in a protective sac).

Omphalocele and gastroschisis require immediate intervention to prevent contamination, followed by repair of the defect.

Assessment

Frequently encountered data for inguinal or imbilical hernia include the following:

Subjective
• colicky abdominal pain
• caregivers' complaint of a "lump" in the child's abdomen

Objective
• inguinal or periumbilical swelling
• palpable mass in abdomen (midline) or groin.

Nursing diagnosis

Potential for Infection related to postoperative wound contamination

Desired outcome: The child is free of wound infection as evidenced by absence of fever, no evidence of inflammation around the incision or wound drainage (or both), and a white blood cell count within normal limits.

Interventions
1. Take appropriate measures to prevent urine or fecal contamination of wound.
2. Fold the child's diaper to ensure it does not contact the wound.
3. Cleanse the surrounding skin area with soap and water; keep the area dry.
4. Maintain a wound cover (may be a collodion dressing or sterile tape).
5. Position the child on his side (not abdomen) during the first 48 hours after surgery.

6. Monitor the child for signs and symptoms of infection.
7. If infection is present, administer antibiotics, as ordered, and monitor for therapeutic effects.

Medical diagnosis

The medical diagnosis for hernia is based on:
• clinical findings
• inspection and palpation.

Medical treatment

Treatment involves surgically repairing the hernia, possibly on an outpatient basis.

Hirschprung's disease

Also known as congenital megacolon, Hirschprung's disease refers to a mechanical obstruction of the bowel caused by the absence or marked reduction of autonomic parasympathetic ganglion cells in a segment of the bowel wall, most commonly the rectosigmoid colon. The length of affected bowel varies. Because of the lack of peristalsis, contents are not propelled forward and bowel obstruction and distention may occur.

Hirschprung's disease, which is more common among boys, may cause enterocolitis and intestinal obstruction. Enterocolitis, which sometimes occurs without diarrhea, may be evident at first by fever and poor feeding in the infant. If not recognized and properly treated, enterocolitis may lead to endotoxic shock.

Assessment

Frequently encountered data for Hirschprungs's disease include the following:

Subjective

• history of vomiting, diarrhea, or constipation

Objective

• The following signs and symptoms vary according to age:
—Newborn: failure to pass meconium, abdominal distention, and vomiting
—Infancy: constipation, abdominal distention, occasional episodes of diarrhea and vomiting
—Childhood: same symptoms as infancy except that stool is ribbonlike and foul-smelling
• palpable fecal masses
• malnutrition and anemia.

Nursing diagnosis

Altered Bowel Elimination: Constipation (Preoperatively) related to effects of anatomic defect
Desired outcome: The child has improved elimination as evidenced by evacuation of stool, a less distended abdomen, less fussiness and irritability, and improved food intake.

Interventions
1. Administer enemas several hours before or after meals, following these guidelines for the usual amount of solution to administer:
• Infant: 150 to 250 ml
• Small child: 250 to 350 ml
• Large child: 300 to 500 ml
• Adolescent: 500 to 700 ml.
2. Teach the caregivers how to administer an enema properly, including information on the preparation of normal saline solution (1 teaspoon of salt to 500 ml of tap water), quantity of solution to administer, and the method of administration.
3. Explain the importance of a low-residue diet and which foods to avoid feeding the child (such as those included in a high-residue diet).
4. Clean the anal area and buttocks and change diapers frequently to prevent excoriation and minimize foul odors.

Nursing diagnosis
Impaired Skin Integrity related to irritating fecal drainage from surgical wound (bowel diversion surgery)
Desired outcome: The child has no evidence of irritation on skin surrounding the stoma.

Interventions
1. Change postoperative wound dressings often; pin or tape a diaper away from the dressing to prevent urine contamination from absorption.
2. Prevent peristomal irritation and breakdown by using a protective appliance.
3. Change or empty the colostomy appliance carefully to avoid irritating the skin.
4. Prevent feces from contacting the skin. If fecal contact occurs, cleanse the skin thoroughly with mild soap and water.
5. Encourage the caregivers to begin providing care for the infant in the hospital to help them gain competence and confidence and thereby develop a sense of control.

Medical diagnosis
The medical diagnosis is based on:
• the patient history
• rectal examination
• barium enema
• rectal biopsy from microscopic examination of cells (may be complicated by enterocolitis).

Medical treatment
Conservative treatment includes:
• daily or more frequent isotonic enemas (of a volume greater than usual for the child's age)
• stool softeners

• digital removal of feces from the rectum
• modification of the child's diet (low-residue diet).
  Surgical intervention includes:
• creation of either a temporary loop or double-barrel colostomy, depending on the child's age
• complete correction at age 1½ to 2, involving removal of the aganglionic bowel and a pull-through procedure
• anastomosis of the intact bowel near the rectum
• closure of the colostomy.

Intussusception

An intestinal obstruction caused by the telescoping of adjacent parts of the bowel, intussusception occurs most frequently in boys under age 2. Children with celiac disease or cystic fibrosis are at increased risk for developing intussusception.

Incarceration commonly occurs at the ileocecal valve. If uncorrected, this obstructed area may develop necrosis with hemorrhage, perforation, and peritonitis.

Assessment

Frequently encountered data for intussusception include:

Subjective
• development of acute abdominal pain in a healthy, thriving child (usually age 3 to 12 months)

Objective
• screaming and drawing knees to chest (with periods of remission)
• progressive vomiting (bile-stained and possibly fecal)
• red, currant jelly–like stools (containing blood and mucus)
• distended and tender abdomen
• fever and prostration (indicating peritonitis).

Nursing diagnosis

Altered Bowel Elimination: (specify problem) related to the development of paralytic ileus secondary to abdominal surgery
Desired outcome: The child recovers from paralytic ileus as evidenced by the presence of bowel sounds, passage of flatus, and relief of abdominal distention.

Interventions
1. Increase the child's activity, as allowed and tolerated (including turning and range-of-motion exercises).
2. Monitor nasogastric tube placement and I.V. fluid infusion to maintain fluid balance.
3. Monitor for signs and symptoms of peritonitis.
4. Comfort the infant who can receive nothing by mouth by providing a pacifier (unless contraindicated by doctor's orders) or holding him.

5. Monitor for return of bowel sounds, relief of distention, and flatus.
6. Begin oral feedings, as ordered.

Nursing diagnosis
Altered Comfort: Pain related to effects of bowel incarceration
Desired outcome: The child's pain diminishes as a result of accurate diagnosis and appropriate treatment.

Interventions
1. Assist in establishing diagnoses by carefully listening to and accurately reporting the caregivers' description of the child's symptoms.
2. Enlist the caregivers' assistance in relieving the child's anxiety and pain by providing information and support.
3. Monitor I.V. fluids and nasogastric suction.
4. Prepare the child for barium enema or surgical intervention, as necessary.
5. Comfort the child by holding, rocking, and stroking him.

Medical diagnosis
A favorable prognosis depends on early detection and treatment. Diagnosis is based on:
• the patient history and physical assessment findings
• barium enema (dangerous if peritonitis has occurred).

Medical treatment
Treatment includes:
• barium enema (may alleviate telescoping)
• surgical intervention to reduce telescoping manually and resect the nonviable intestine.

Malabsorption syndrome
A group of symptoms resulting from impaired intestinal absorption of nutrients, malabsorption syndrome may be caused by digestive, absorptive, or anatomical defects. For example, in cystic fibrosis, a digestive defect caused by the absence of a digestive enzyme results in malabsorption of nutrients.

Impairment of the mucosal transport system may be caused by a primary defect (such as celiac disease, the most common defect) or may be secondary to another disorder (such as ulcerative colitis, which results in accelerated motility, and Hirschsprung's disease with enterocolitis, an obstructive disorder).

Structural defects, such as short-bowel syndrome, that occur after extensive resection of the digestive tract decrease the time available for nutrient absorption.

Assessment
Signs and symptoms vary with the underlying cause. Celiac disease, the most common defect in children, may have a familial tendency. Associated with an intolerance to gluten, this disease

results in the destruction of small-intestine villi when gluten is consumed in the diet. When progressively exposed to gluten, the intestine cannot absorb nutrients.

Objective data
- steatorrhea (fat, foul, frothy, watery stools)
- general malnutrition (characterized by muscle wasting, abdominal distention, behavioral changes, vitamin deficiencies, anemia, constipation, vomiting, and abdominal pain)

Nursing diagnosis
Altered Nutrition: Less Than Body Requirements related to effects of damage to the absorptive surfaces of the small intestine caused by gluten
Desired outcome: The child has a weight gain of (specify amount) _____lb within (specify time) _____.

Interventions
1. Explain to the caregivers the disease process and the role gluten plays in the disorder.
2. Provide dietary restrictions for gluten, including the elimination of wheat, rye, barley, and oats from the child's diet.
3. Encourage careful assessment for gluten in the ingredients of prepared foods.
4. Stress the use of gluten-free grains, such as rice and corn.
5. Allow the caregivers to express feelings related to increased expenses of alternative diets and the difficulty in ensuring the child's adherence to the regimen.
6. Reaffirm the benefits of the diet to the child's growth and development.
7. As the child reaches an age for self-care, include him in explanations about the importance of life-long nutritional limitations.

Nursing diagnosis
Fluid Volume Deficit related to dehydration and metabolic acidosis secondary to celiac crisis precipitated by infection, dietary glutens, or anticholinergic crisis
Desired outcome: The child's fluid balance is restored.

Interventions
1. Assess the child for signs and symptoms of metabolic acidosis, including decreasing level of consciousness, irritability, weakness, and irregular pulse.
2. Assess for signs and symptoms of dehydration.
3. Monitor intake and output closely. (Measure nasogastric tube drainage and I.V. fluids carefully to determine exact intake and output.)
4. Provide good mouth and skin care to maintain integrity.
5. Counsel the caregivers on preventive care measures, such as good health maintenance, dietary control, and avoidance of harmful medications.

Medical diagnosis
The medical diagnosis for malabsorption syndrome caused by celiac disease is based on:
• the patient history
• clinical manifestations (usually do not appear until after age 1 when child begins ingesting foods that contain gluten)
• stool analysis
• hematologic studies (to indicate deficiencies)
• peroral jejunal biopsy (by way of a tube passed through the mouth to the jejunum)
• clinical improvement after institution of a gluten-restricted diet.

Medical treatment
Treatment includes the following:
• gluten-restricted diet
• replacement of deficient nutrients, including vitamins and iron
• prompt intervention to correct dehydration.

Hypertrophic pyloric stenosis
A congenital defect characterized by obstruction of the pylorus of the stomach, hypertrophic pyloric stenosis occurs more commonly among boys. Evident soon after birth, this condition is marked by vomiting that becomes progressively more severe and projectile. Possibly hereditary, this disorder results from hypertrophy of the circular muscle surrounding the pylorus. As the muscle thickens, the stomach usually dilates. Inflammation and edema cause a partial obstruction of the pyloric orifice to become further obstructed, sometimes resulting in complete obstruction.

Assessment
Frequently encountered data for hypertrophic pyloric stenosis include the following:

Subjective
• history of vomiting

Objective
• regurgitation and nonprojectile vomiting beginning at age 2 to 4 weeks that develops into projectile vomiting (ejected 2' to 4' shortly after feeding)
• resultant dehydration (characterized by sunken eyeballs and loss of tissue turgor)
• failure to gain weight or loss of weight
• upper abdominal distention
• "olive" sign (presence of a palpable pyloric sphincter)
• visible left-to-right peristaltic waves.

Nursing diagnosis
Altered Nutrition: Less Than Body Requirements related to eme-

sis or postoperative status
Desired outcome: The child retains food, maintains hydration, and gains weight.

Interventions
1. Give the child small, frequent, thickened feedings, as ordered.
2. Feed the child slowly.
3. Bubble (burp) the child before, during, and after feeding.
4. Place the child on his right side in Fowler's position after feeding.
5. Handle the child sparingly and gently after feeding.

Nursing diagnosis
Altered Comfort: Pain related to unsatisfactory feeding event
Desired outcome: The infant appears more satisfied as evidenced by a reduction in crying and restlessness.

Interventions
1. Provide a pacifier to meet the child's oral needs when he can receive nothing by mouth.
2. Encourage caregivers to visit and assist with care, when appropriate.
3. Hold and stroke the infant between feedings.
4. Administer medications for postoperative pain, as ordered.

Medical diagnosis
The medical diagnosis for hypertrophic pyloric stenosis is based on:
• clinical signs and symptoms related by the caregivers
• palpable pyloric mass
• upper GI studies
• evaluation of metabolic alteration through serum electrolyte studies.

Medical treatment
Nonsurgical interventions include:
• use of a thickened formula
• small, frequent feedings
• administration of cholinergic blockers.
   Surgical interventions include:
• initial rehydration followed by correction of metabolic alterations
• pylorotomy (has a high success rate)
• postoperative feedings every 4 to 6 hours; small amounts of glucose and electrolytes in water are given for 24 hours in step-by-step increments until formula is tolerated at full feeding schedule (usually in about 48 hours).

Ulcerative colitis
Ulcerative colitis, an inflammatory bowel disease involving the mucosa and submucosa of the large intestine, occurs in all age-

groups; however, peak incidence in children occurs between ages 10 and 19. Although the exact etiology is unknown, this disorder is believed to be organic, caused by a combination of infections and nutritional, immunologic, and psychogenic factors.

Characteristically, the mucous membranes of the bowel become hyperemic and edematous and eventually ulcerate. Over time, the lumen of the bowel narrows and smoothes, resulting in a thinned or absent mucosal lining with a greatly reduced absorptive area.

Ulcerative colitis may categorized as follows:
• acute, remitting colitis, characterized by remissions and exacerbations (may respond to medical treatment)
• chronic, continuous colitis, characterized by chronic malnutrition and anemia (responds poorly to treatment).

Assessment
Frequently encountered data for ulcerative colitis include the following:

Subjective
• cramping
• abdominal pain

Objective
• persistent, recurring diarrhea (marked by urgency, frequency, and possible bloodiness)
• fever
• weight loss, anorexia, and nausea and vomiting
• anemia
• electrolyte imbalance.

Nursing diagnosis
Altered Nutrition: Less Than Body Requirements related to inadequate oral intake or decreased absorption of nutrients
Desired outcome: The child gains weight and approaches his normal level, has increased strength and activity tolerance, and has laboratory values within normal ranges.

Interventions
1. Monitor the therapeutic and adverse effects of total parenteral nutrition (generally the reason for hospitalization).
2. Assess for signs and symptoms of fluid imbalances, including:
• altered intake and output
• changes in specific gravity, skin turgor, and vital signs
• low blood pressure
• increased pulse rate
• electrolyte imbalance.
3. Take the following measures to improve the child's oral intake (when allowed):
• Provide oral care before meals.
• Feed small portions of appealing food.

• Promote a quiet, relaxed atmosphere during meals.
4. Reassess the child's nutritional status every 72 hours, using calorie counts and daily weights.
5. Assess for therapeutic and adverse effects of medications, including vitamin and mineral supplements.

Nursing diagnosis
Altered Bowel Elimination: Diarrhea related to intestinal hyperactivity
Desired outcome: The child has fewer bowel movements and more formed stool.

Interventions
1. Assess bowel sounds and the frequency of bowel movements.
2. Rest the child's bowel by maintaining fluid and food restrictions and promoting rest.
3. When the child is allowed oral intake, provide information on nutrients; also, add one new food at a time and give small, frequent meals.
4. Monitor the child for therapeutic and adverse effects of corticosteroids, antispasmodics, antibacterials, and bulk-forming agents.

Nursing diagnosis
Altered Comfort related to abdominal cramping and pain, anorectal pain, or oral pain (specify) secondary to membrane lesions
Desired outcome: The child's pain diminishes as evidenced by his reports of decreased pain and relaxed body language.

Interventions
1. Assess the child for verbal and nonverbal communication of pain.
2. Wash and dry the anal area thoroughly after each bowel movement and sitz bath.
3. Provide an anorectal anesthetic, as ordered.
4. Use a soft brush and low-pressure mouth irrigation when providing mouth care.
5. Avoid feeding the child hot, spicy, or acidic foods.
6. Use appropriate measures to relieve pain, such as position changes, relaxation techniques, and distraction.

Medical diagnosis
The medical diagnosis for ulcerative colitis is based on:
• the patient history
• barium enema revealing a "lead-pipe" colon (marked by loss of a normal scalloped appearance and a consistently decreased diameter)
• rectosigmoidoscopy
• mucosal biopsy
• stool and blood studies.

Medical treatment

Treatment during an acute episode includes:

• hospitalization (to ensure disease management and eliminate possible environmental factors)

• total parenteral nutrition (to allow the colon to rest and to improve nutritional status)

• administration of medication (to reduce abdominal pain and rectal spasm)

• administration of steroids (to reduce bowel inflammation)

• administration of antibacterial medication, such as sulfasalazine (to alleviate or prevent infection).

Surgical intervention involves temporary colostomy or total colostomy with a permanent ileostomy.

☐ Genitourinary and reproductive systems

Within this section, you'll find a discussion of diseases and disorders affecting reproduction and the genitourinary system. Some anomalies of the genitourinary system may be apparent at birth; others may not be diagnosed until the impact on excretory function provokes a systemic response. Early diagnosis and treatment enable a child with such a disease or disorder to maintain renal function as near to normal as possible.

Because of the lifelong threats to self-image and satisfaction of sexual needs, cosmetic and reproductive deficits require correction early in childhood. The overwhelming psychosocial implications of such genitourinary problems present a special challenge to the nurse, especially in regard to the child's and caregivers' ability to cope with the situation.

Admission assessment

During your assessment, ask the caregivers or child (as appropriate) the following questions to obtain a comprehensive genitourinary and reproductive history:

Patient history. Find out about the following:

• Urinary function: Does the child cry or complain of pain or burning when voiding? Does the child feel urgency? Does he feel the need to urinate frequently? How much and how frequently does he void? Is he toilet-trained? At what age was he trained? Has he had any regression? Does he have nocturia or enuresis? Does he have a fever? Has there been a change in urine color? Does the urine have any unusual odor? Has the child ever been treated for a urinary tract infection?

• Pain: Does the child have any evidence of flank, suprapubic, or back pain?

• Swelling: Does the child's face look puffy, especially in the morning? Has any swelling of hands or feet been noted? Has the child experienced any recent weight gain?

• Itching: Has the child been scratching the perianal area?

• Discharge: Has there been any vaginal or penile discharge? (If so, have the caregivers or child describe the color, odor, consistency, and amount.)

• Lesions: Does the child have any rashes, sores, ulcers, or blisters in the urethral or genital area? (If so, have the caregivers or child describe the location and size.) Has the child been exposed to any sexually transmitted diseases?

• Menstrual history: At what age did the child reach menarche? How long and how frequently do menses occur? Does she experience any menstrual pain, dysmenorrhea, metrorrhagia, or menorrhagia? Is she sexually active? Has she ever been pregnant? (If so, obtain a detailed history of the pregnancy.) What method of birth control does she use?

• Allergies: Is the child allergic to iodine? (Ask about this because contrast media for diagnostic studies may contain iodine.)

Family history. Ask about a family history of renal failure, diabetes mellitus, hypertension, renal calculi, and anomalies, such as epispadias, hypospadias, cryptorchidism, polycystic kidneys, and renal tumors. Also ask whether the child was exposed to diethylstilbestrol (DES) before birth.

Physical assessment
During the physical assessment, be sure to check the child's vital signs, including blood pressure. Also, measure and chart the height and weight (see the "Physical Growth Charts" in the Appendices).

Skin. Assess skin color for pallor, which is characteristic of anemia caused by renal failure. A child with renal failure may have rough, dry, scaly skin with evidence of scratch marks. Evaluate skin turgor for evidence of dehydration or edema.

Cardiovascular status. A systolic murmur may point to anemia from renal failure. Changes in heart rate or rhythm may indicate fluid or electrolyte imbalance.

Respiratory status. Auscultate the lungs for evidence of fluid overload.

Abdomen. Auscultate for bowel sounds. Palpate for bladder distention, ascites, masses, and tenderness.

Kidneys. With the child sitting, palpate the kidneys for size and tenderness, then auscultate for bruits. With the child supine, perform bimanual palpation, then percuss the flanks to assess for pain.

Genitalia. Depending on the child's sex, assess for the following:
Female genitalia
• Mons pubis: Inspect for skin discoloration, hair distribution, and pubic lice. Palpate for masses.

• Clitoris: Inspect for size and position; however, avoid palpation because the clitoris is extremely sensitive. Keep in mind that an abnormally large clitoris may be an ambiguous small penis.
• Labia majora: Observe for lesions or inflammation. Palpate for labioinguinal hernia. Keep in mind that fused labia may be an ambiguous small scrotum.
• Bartholin's and Skene's glands: These should not be visible or palpable.
• Labia minora: Inspect for adhesions and hygiene. Keep in mind that the labia minora are prominent in the newborn.
• Urinary meatus: Inspect for inflammation or discharge. Take cultures of discharge, if ordered.
• Vaginal orifice: Inspect for patency, signs of irritation, discharge, or the possibility of foreign body insertion. Note any foul smell. Take cultures of discharge, if ordered.

Male genitalia
• Testes: Check for undescended testes. Be sure your hands are warm, as cold hands will stimulate the cremasteric reflex and retract the testicle. Use soap or lotion to lubricate your fingers and to avoid traumatizing the child. Block the inguinal canal with your opposite hand to trap the testicle in the scrotal sac.

If you cannot palpate the testicle, try palpating with the child in a squatting position with his legs crossed in front of him or sitting in a chair with his knees drawn up against his chest. Position an infant supine with his legs raised and spread.

Palpate the testes for symmetry and smoothness. Skin should be rugose. If the scrotal sac is smooth and small with midline separation and the testes cannot be palpated, this may be enlarged labia of ambiguous genitalia.
• Scrotum: Assess for edema, inflammation, lesions, and masses. If the child has a suspected hydrocele, transillumination may be used to rule out other problems. Keep in mind that the scrotum may normally hang slightly lower on one side.
• Penis: The penis should be at least 1″ long in a newborn. If less than 1″, the child may have an ambiguous clitoris. (*Note:* Never retract the foreskin of an infant under age 4 months.) Observe for inflammation and edema. Note the position and size of the urinary meatus. Look for lesions or ulceration. Inspect for size and patency of foreskin (in uncircumcised children).

Urine specimen. Usually, the child will need to produce a urine specimen during the admission and assessment process. Keep the following points in mind:
• Explain to the caregivers or child (if appropriate) why the specimen is needed.
• If the child is toilet-trained, enlist his help in obtaining the specimen. Respect the child's desire to do it alone (if old enough) or to have his caregivers help.
• Use vocabulary familiar to the child.

• Demonstrate how to obtain the specimen using the necessary equipment (wipes and container).
• Emphasize the need to avoid contaminating the equipment.
• Wait at least 30 minutes after the child's last voiding before attempting to collect urine.
• If the child is not toilet-trained, use a U bag (see *Using a U bag,* pages 152 and 153).
• If a sterile specimen is required, you may need to catheterize the child or assist with a suprapubic tap (see *Assisting with a suprapubic tap,* page 155).

Bladder extrophy

Bladder extrophy, a relatively rare but serious congenital defect involving absence of the lower abdominal wall and anterior bladder wall and eversion of the posterior bladder wall, occurs more often in boys.

Assessment

An obvious congenital defect, this disorder often is accompanied by other, less obvious anomalies.

Nursing diagnosis

Potential for Infection (Urinary Tract) related to the effects of exposure of ureteral orifices
Desired outcome: The child has no evidence of renal damage.

Interventions

1. Apply sterile petrolatum gauze over the defect, then place absorbent diapers over the gauze.
2. Administer prophylactic antibiotics or urinary antiseptics, as ordered.
3. Provide sponge baths only; do not immerse the child in water to bathe him.
4. Assess for signs and symptoms of infection, including fever and cloudy, foul-smelling urine.
5. Maintain good hydration.

Nursing diagnosis

Impaired Skin Integrity related to constant exposure to urine
Desired outcome: The child has no evidence of skin ulceration or infection.

Interventions

Change all dressings and diapers frequently to keep the child's skin as clean and dry as possible.

Nursing diagnosis

Urinary Incontinence related to the effects of bladder anomaly
Desired outcome: The child attains urinary continence.

(continued on page 154)

USING A U BAG

Debra Lister, your 8-month-old patient, has the signs and symptoms of a urinary infection. To confirm the diagnosis, the doctor's ordered a urine culture. But how can you collect a specimen from a child who's not yet toilet-trained?

Chances are, you'll collect a specimen with a U bag (urine collection bag). This noninvasive plastic device fits temporarily over the child's perineal area, capturing urine as she excretes it. Some models have a nonreflux flap to prevent urine from escaping. To learn how to collect a specimen using a U bag, read on.

1

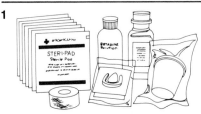

Collect the equipment shown here: a U bag, nine 4" x 4" sterile gauze pads (or cotton balls), antimicrobial solution, sterile normal saline solution or water, and a sterile specimen container with lid. To help secure the bag, also obtain 1" (2.5-cm) nonallergenic tape.

Nursing tip: Unless contraindicated, give the child something to drink 30 minutes before performing the procedure. This helps ensure adequate urine production.

Thoroughly wash your hands. Open all of the sterile gauze pads. Moisten three of them with antimicrobial solution, and three with sterile saline solution. Let the other three remain dry. Make sure all your equipment's within easy reach.

2

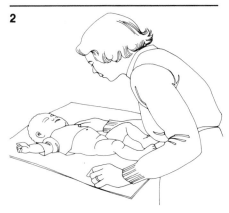

Place the child in a supine position, and remove her diaper. Even though she's too young to understand an explanation of the procedure, remember to speak soothingly to her, as the nurse is doing here.

Important: If Debra's parents are present, tell them why the specimen's needed, and describe the cleansing and collection procedures. Assure them that the procedure's not painful, but that the child may find the bag uncomfortable or annoying. Tell them that you'll remove the bag as soon as enough urine has accumulated (usually within 20 minutes).

3

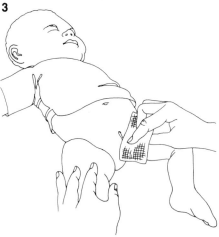

Now, prepare to cleanse Debra's perineal area. First, position Debra with her legs apart, as shown here, and separate her labia. Using one of the pads moistened with antimicrobial solution, gently cleanse one side of the labia, as the nurse is doing in this illustration. Cleanse from front to back, to avoid fecal contamination. Discard the gauze pad and repeat the procedure on the other side of the labia, using another pad moistened in antimicrobial solution. Finally, take the last of these pads, and cleanse the urethral opening. To prevent irritation, rinse her perineal area with the gauze pads soaked in sterile saline solution. Follow the same procedure as for cleansing.

Then, use the dry gauze pads to dry the perineum. This step reduces the risk of skin chapping and allows the adhesive strip to stick securely to her skin.

4

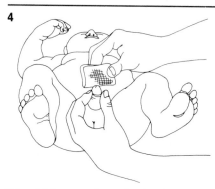

If the child's an uncircumcised male, pull back his foreskin. Then, take a wipe moistened with antimicrobial solution and begin cleansing the head of the penis, working from the urethral opening toward his abdomen. Discard the wipe after one stroke. Repeat the cleansing procedure with each of the remaining two wipes, discarding each wipe after one use. Rinse the penis, following the same procedure as for cleansing, and dry the area.

5

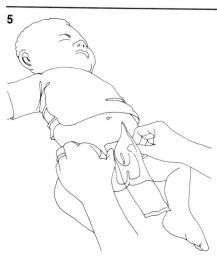

Remove the paper backing from the U bag's top adhesive strip. Then, center the bag's opening over the child's labia, and press the adhesive firmly in place. When the bag's

properly centered, remove the U bag's bottom adhesive strip, and firmly press this adhesive in place, too. Smooth out any loose edges or bubbles in the adhesive strips. For added security, consider reinforcing them with a strip of 1″ (2.5-cm) nonallergenic tape.

If your patient's a boy, place his penis inside the bag, and firmly press the backing against his skin. Reinforce the adhesive with nonallergenic tape, if necessary.

Unless contraindicated, place the child in semi-Fowler's position to facilitate drainage into the bag. Give her a toy to play with or ask her parents to distract her, if she's active.

Nursing tip: If you apply a diaper over the bag, allow the bottom of the bag to protrude from the diaper, so you can check urine accumulation.

6

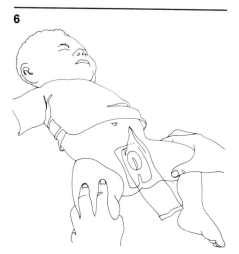

Check the bag at least every 15 minutes to assess urine production. As soon as about 20 ml of urine accumulates, remove the bag. By removing the bag as soon as possible, you reduce the risk that it'll loosen, which may spill or contaminate the specimen.

Note: If the infant doesn't urinate within 30 minutes, remove the bag, prep her perineal area again, and apply a new bag. This precaution minimizes the risk of specimen contamination.

Pour the urine specimen into the sterile specimen container, and cover it securely with the lid. Label the container, and send it to the lab at once. Properly dispose of the U bag and other soiled equipment. Wash your hands, and document the procedure.

Interventions

1. Provide extensive preoperative and postoperative physical and psychological care of the child. (Numerous surgeries may be required.)
2. Involve the family in caring for the child during his hospitalization. (This will ease them into home management.)

Nursing diagnosis

Ineffective Individual and Family Coping related to the inability to deal with bladder anomaly and incontinence
Desired outcome: The family (and later, the child) use available resources for correction and long-term management.

Interventions

1. Provide extensive preoperative and postoperative physical and psychological care. (Numerous surgeries may be required.)
2. Involve the caregivers and other family members in caring for the child during his hospitalization. (This will ease them into home management.)
3. See "Epispadias and hypospadias" in this section for interventions regarding caregiver bonding.

Nursing diagnosis

Impaired Physical Mobility: Gait Disturbance related to separation of the pubic bones
Desired outcome: The child has a normal gait after intervention.

Interventions

1. Provide usual nursing care measures for the child in a brace.
2. Provide preoperative and postoperative care if surgery is required.
3. Assist the family in understanding the treatment to help improve compliance.
4. Teach the family how to care for the child with an appliance or brace to prevent complications.

Medical diagnosis

Although the defect is obvious at birth, thorough assessment is required to determine associated skeletal malfunctions.

Medical treatment

Treatment aims to:
• achieve urinary control
• maintain renal function
• obtain a satisfactory cosmetic result
• promote satisfactory sexual and psychological outcomes.

Surgery provides closure of the defect or urinary diversion, enabling the child to enjoy socialization and childhood activities. Reconstruction may involve several stages. The child and caregiv-

ASSISTING WITH A SUPRAPUBIC TAP

You've been trying to collect a urine specimen from 13-month-old Kevin Borelli. But because he has diaper rash, the bag's adhesive strip won't stick firmly to his skin. What's more, Kevin's becoming increasingly upset as the bag irritates his already-inflamed skin. To spare Kevin prolonged discomfort, the doctor's ordered a suprapubic tap.

As you probably know, a suprapubic tap allows the doctor to obtain a sterile urine specimen. Although it's an invasive procedure, a suprapubic tap carries fewer risks of infection or trauma than does catheterization. What's your role? To find out, read the following.

1 Gather the sterile equipment you'll need: a 20-ml syringe, a 20G or 21G 14″ needle, a specimen container, and a 4″ x 4″ gauze pad. In addition, obtain a patient label for the specimen container, a povidone-iodine preparation, and an alcohol wipe.

Unless contraindicated, offer Kevin fluids before the procedure to help ensure adequate urine production. Inform the doctor if Kevin's urinated within the past hour. The doctor will probably postpone the procedure until the bladder has time to fill again.

2 Before the doctor begins the procedure, speak soothingly to Kevin so he's as quiet as possible. But if your patient's an older child, provide a simple explanation of the procedure. For example, tell him that the doctor will prick his tummy, and that it will hurt. But emphasize that the discomfort will last only a very short time, and tell the child that he can help you and the doctor by holding as still as possible.

3

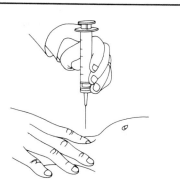

Now, undress the child, place him supine on an exam table, and restrain him with his legs spread apart. Or, grasp both his feet in one hand, and draw them toward his body. Speak reassuringly to the child throughout the procedure.

While the child's restrained, the doctor will palpate his bladder and cleanse the puncture site.

Before the doctor aspirates the specimen, he may ask you to apply pressure to the child's urethra. If necessary, ask a co-worker to restrain the child. Then, gently squeeze the penis, to occlude the urethra. (If your patient's a girl, apply direct pressure on her urethra or apply upward pressure through her rectum.) Then, the doctor will insert the needle into the bladder, as shown, and aspirate a urine specimen.

4

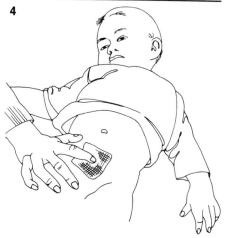

As soon as the doctor removes the needle, apply gentle pressure over the puncture site with the sterile gauze pad. As you do, comfort and praise your patient. After bleeding stops, dress him and make him as comfortable as possible. An older child may want you to put a colorful adhesive bandage strip over the puncture site.

Eject the urine specimen from the syringe into the sterile container, label the container, and send it to the lab at once. Document the procedure in your nurses' notes.

Important: Following the procedure, observe the child for hematuria (bloody urine). Document any blood traces you see, and notify the doctor immediately if bleeding is prolonged or seems excessive.

ers need honest information to avoid any unrealistic expectations of the final results of treatment.

Cryptorchidism

Common in premature infants and children with cystic fibrosis, cryptorchidism refers to failure of the testes to descend from the abdominal cavity (where they develop in utero) into the scrotal sac. Normally, this descent occurs during the 7th to 9th month of gestation.

Cryptorchidism, which can be unilateral or bilateral, occurs one of two ways:
• the testicle never descends from the abdominal cavity
• the testicle begins descending but lodges in the perineum or thigh.

Assessment

This condition is discovered during the initial neonatal examination; the child is observed for spontaneous descent during subsequent visits.

Nursing diagnosis

Sexual Dysfunction: Infertility related to the effects of testicular damage
Desired outcome: The child's testes are located in the scrotal sac before irreversible damage to spermatogenic function occurs.

Interventions

1. Assist with preoperative preparation and postoperative care of the child undergoing orchiopexy. (In this procedure, the testicle is brought down into the scrotal sac and maintained in position with a traction suture.)
2. Note the following special postoperative nursing considerations:
• Apply ice packs, if ordered, to reduce edema.
• Provide scrupulous cleansing of the perineum to prevent fecal contamination of the suture line.
• Use caution to avoid disturbing the tension mechanism.
• Administer antibiotics, as ordered, to prevent infection.

Nursing diagnosis

Disturbance in Self-concept: Altered Body Image related to absence of testicle in the scrotal sac
Desired outcome: The child does not verbalize evidence of a disturbed body image.

Interventions

1. If the testicle is totally absent or must be removed, a prosthesis may be implanted in the scrotal sac to give a normal appearance.
2. See Section 4 for specific care measures.

Medical diagnosis

The medical diagnosis for cryptorchidism is based on the physical assessment.

Medical treatment

Treatment aims to prevent infertility and testicular cancer and to obtain a normal cosmetic appearance. (Implant of a prosthesis usually is scheduled before the child begins school.) This condition may be managed on an outpatient basis with the administration of chorionic gonadotropin hormone.

Epispadias and hypospadias

Congenital conditions in which the urinary meatus opens in an abnormal position, epispadias and hypospadias occur in both boys and girls but more commonly in boys.

In epispadias, the urethra opens on the dorsal surface of the penis or a fissure is present the rostral wall of the female urethra. In hypospadias, the urethra opens on the underside of the penis or in the vagina. In boys, hypospadias commonly is associated with congenital chordee, a condition involving downward bowing of the penis.

These defects occur in varying degrees. In some cases, the deformity is so minimal that no treatment is required. In other cases, the deformity may be so severe that the child's gender cannot be determined.

Assessment

Epispadias and hypospadias are detected soon after birth by medical or nursing staff. Nurses working in newborn nurseries are responsible for assessing infant voiding patterns and should report any observed defects.

Nursing diagnosis

Altered Parenting: Ineffective Bonding related to disappointment in the physical characteristics of the child and interruption of the bonding process by hospitalization
Desired outcome: The caregivers verbalize understanding and acceptance of the child and demonstrate attachment behaviors.

Interventions

1. Support the caregivers through the process of understanding the condition, its significance, and the plan of treatment. (Early hospitalization may be required to release a chordee, but further reconstructive surgery usually is delayed.)
2. Create an environment that invites and welcomes caregiver participation.

Nursing diagnosis

Altered Family Process (Jewish) related to necessity for delay of circumcision

Desired outcome: The family verbalizes resolution of the conflict between practicing their Jewish faith and adhering to the current treatment plan. (*Note:* Circumcision usually is delayed so that the prepuce skin can be saved for future reconstructive surgery. Reconstructive surgery may be delayed until the penis is large enough.)

Interventions

1. Carefully explain to the family the reason why circumcision will be delayed.
2. Enlist the help of supportive clergy if a religious circumcision was planned.

Nursing diagnosis

Disturbance in Self-concept: Altered Body Image related to fear of castration or mutilation

Desired outcome: The child and family acknowledge and discuss fears about possible body changes, and the child develops a positive body image.

Interventions

1. Apply general principles of pediatric preoperative and postoperative care (see Section 4).
2. Provide information, support, and psychological preparation for surgery. (Ideally, surgery is planned when the penis is large enough but before the child reaches an age when he fears mutilation.)
3. Be alert for indications of fear, such as denial or depression.
4. Deal with the child's and caregivers' expectations in an honest, realistic manner.

Medical diagnosis

The medical diagnosis for epispadias and hypospadias is based on:
• radiographic studies using contrast media (may be used to determine the extent of the anomaly and the urine pathway)
• chromosomal studies (may be required in severe cases to determine the infant's gender).

Medical treatment

Treatment aims to:
• promote psychological well-being via satisfactory cosmetic results
• direct the urine stream in the normal fashion
• construct a sexually adequate organ.

Depending on the degree of involvement, several surgical procedures may be required to achieve adequate results. Ideally, all surgery is completed before the child starts school.

Glomerulonephritis, acute

The most common renal disease affecting children, acute glomerulo-nephritis (AGN) accounts for approximately 0.5% of all pediatric hospital admissions. AGN affects boys twice as often as girls, with peak incidence in children occurring between ages 2 and 12.

An immunologic disorder secondary to an infection elsewhere in the body, AGN usually is associated with group A beta-hemolytic streptococcal infection of the upper respiratory tract or skin. Other possible causative microorganisms include pneumococci, staphylococci, mumps virus, varicella virus, and Epstein-Barr virus.

AGN is marked by immune complexes deposited in the glomeruli, decreased glomerular filtration rate, and hypervolemia with edema. Renal symptoms usually occur about 3 to 4 weeks after onset of the primary infection. The prognosis is excellent with prompt and adequate treatment.

Assessment

Frequently encountered data for AGN include the following:

Subjective (as reported by the caregiver)
• cola-colored urine
• oliguria
• fever
• puffy eyes
• vomiting
• diarrhea
• headache

Objective
• hematuria
• elevated urine specific gravity
• periorbital edema
• hypertension (in about two thirds of affected children).

Nursing diagnosis

Fluid Volume Excess related to decreased glomerular filtration rate
Desired outcome: The child's weight and blood pressure are within normal levels, the child has no evidence of edema, and intake and output are balanced.

Interventions
1. Assess for the following signs and symptoms of fluid overload:
• elevated blood pressure
• bounding pulse
• tachypnea and shallow, labored respirations
• crackles or rhonchi on auscultation
• pitting edema
• distended neck veins (associated with elevated central venous pressure)

• weight gain (as revealed by daily evaluation).

2. Institute the following measures, as ordered, for antihypertensive therapy, including:

• administration of furosemide, reserpine, or hydralazine

• administration of barbiturates

• restriction of fluids during the oliguric phase

• a low-sodium diet (may require creativity to avoid compromising the child's appetite)

• bed rest.

Nursing diagnosis

Potential for Infection related to the high-risk status of the child with AGN

Desired outcome: Interventions destroy the infecting organisms, prevent the occurrence of secondary infection, and shorten the course of the disease.

Interventions

1. Administer antibiotics (usually penicillin), as ordered.

2. Avoid exposing the child to infected individuals.

3. Provide scrupulous skin care.

Nursing diagnosis

Altered Thought Processes related to complications of hypertensive encephalopathy secondary to retained sodium, water, and cerebral vasospasm

Desired outcome: The child has no evidence of altered thought processes as evidenced by assessing the level of consciousness.

Interventions

1. Observe and report the following signs and symptoms of hypertensive encephalopathy

• headache

• drowsiness

• vomiting

• restlessness

• diplopia

• seizures.

2. Institute seizure precautions.

3. Provide prompt and effective management of hypertension.

Medical diagnosis

The medical diagnosis for AGN is based on:

• history of previous infection

• urinalysis (to check for hematuria, proteinuria, elevated specific gravity, and casts)

• elevated antistreptolysin O (ASO) titer

• streptozyme test (more sensitive than ASO titer)

• elevated creatinine and blood urea nitrogen levels (in 50% of cases)

- elevated erythrocyte sedimentation rate and C-reactive protein levels
- chest X-ray showing cardiomegaly and pulmonary edema
- EKG changes.

Medical treatment
Treatment includes supportive care and interventions to treat hypertension to prevent complications of encephalopathy, cardiac failure, or renal failure. Dialysis may be necessary if renal failure occurs.

Nephrosis (nephrotic syndrome)
Nephrosis involves pathologic changes in the glomeruli that result in severe proteinuria, hypoalbuminemia, edema, and hyperlipidemia; nephrosis may be idiopathic, congenital, or secondary to another disease or disorder.

Most cases are idiopathic and primarily occur in boys age 2 to 3. The congenital condition, caused by autosomal recessive transmission, has a poor prognosis. Secondary nephrosis may result from systemic disease or renal disorders, such as acute or chronic glomerulonephritis.

Assessment
Frequently encountered data for nephrosis include the following:

Subjective
- as reported by caregiver:
    —weight gain (may be gradual or sudden)
    —swelling around the eyes in the morning
    —swelling of the feet and ankles later in the day
    —paleness
- nausea, vomiting, and diarrhea
- malaise and anorexia

Objective
- elevated urine specific gravity
- proteinuria
- oliguria
- hepatomegaly
- normal blood pressure and temperature (usually)
- ascites and periorbital edema.

Nursing diagnosis
Fluid Volume Excess related to decreased plasma protein levels
Desired outcome: The child has a stabilized fluid volume, increased urine output, absence of protein from urine, reduced edema, and no discomfort from edema.

Interventions
1. Monitor intake and output accurately to assess progress and

evaluate fluid requirements. (In an infant or toddler, this may require weighing of diapers or underpads.)

2. Provide a diet high in protein and low in sodium. Keep in mind the following dietary considerations:
• Make meals as appetizing as possible.
• Provide small portions.
• Promote a pleasant atmosphere for mealtimes; ask family members or other children to keep the child company during meals.
• Provide the child with his favorite foods, as appropriate.
• Allow foods from home, as appropriate.

3. Weigh the child daily, making sure all weights are accurate by weighing the child in the same clothing at the same time each day, using the same scale.

4. Administer diuretics and steroids, as ordered. (Familiarize yourself with each medication's actions, precautions, and possible adverse effects.)

5. Administer low-sodium albumin I.V., as ordered; carefully monitor the I.V. site and prevent complications.

6. Obtain daily urine specimens for specific gravity and protein levels.

7. Monitor the child's vital signs every 4 hours. (Steroids may elevate blood pressure.) Also, observe for signs and symptoms of respiratory distress.

8. Change the child's position frequently; place him in high Fowler's position if he has respiratory distress.

9. Measure the child's abdominal girth daily. (If paracentesis is ordered, assist the doctor and support and comfort the child.)

10. Assist with ambulation to avoid injury. (Edema may result in unbalanced gait and falls. Bones are susceptible to fracture because of demineralization from steroids.)

11. Carefully monitor a child undergoing chemotherapy. (Immunosuppressive medications, such as chlorambucil and cyclophosphamide, may be used if child does not respond to other modes of treatment.)

Nursing diagnosis

Potential for Infection (especially pneumococcal) related to the effects of debilitated condition and drug therapy
Desired outcome: The child has no evidence of infection.

Interventions

1. Monitor for signs and symptoms of infection.
2. Avoid exposing the child to infected persons.
3. Promote adequate rest to avoid fatigue.
4. Administer antibiotics, as ordered.
5. Report cough, nasal discharge, or other signs and symptoms of upper respiratory tract infection.
6. Use aseptic technique in administering all nursing care.
7. Teach the child good hygienic practices.

8. Take appropriate measures to prevent skin breakdown.

9. Cleanse edematous eyelids with warm sterile saline solution several times each day to remove dried secretions.

10. Assist in obtaining and caring for specimens, as ordered.

Nursing diagnosis

Compromised Family Coping related to the effects of the chronic nature of nephrotic syndrome and lack of preparation for the stress entailed

Desired outcome: The family is actively involved in caring for the child during the hospitalization and demonstrates coping skills as a preparation for discharge.

Interventions

1. Assess the family's ability to cope with previous crisis situations.

2. Provide information and prepare the family for possible outcomes, including:

• spontaneous or therapeutically induced remission without relapse or with repeated relapses

• failure to respond to treatment, chronic illness, and progressive renal disease.

Note: A favorable outcome occurs in 70% to 75% of cases; however, the treatment usually takes 1 to 1½ years. No method for predicting which children will have a favorable outcome exists.

3. Prepare the family for the child's mood swings, which may range from depression and irritability to high spirits; such mood swings are related to the illness and the effect of steroids.

4. Support the caregivers during the child's frequent hospitalizations. Allow them to assist with care; remember to relieve them for rest periods.

5. Prepare for the child's discharge by teaching:

• urine testing

• administration guidelines and adverse effects of medications (when to call the doctor)

• signs of relapse

• the importance of the child's returning to school as soon as possible

• other means of maintaining as normal a life-style as possible.

Medical diagnosis

The medical diagnosis for nephrosis is based on:

• clinical findings

• laboratory values (serum cholesterol level of 300 to 1,800 mg/dl, elevated serum sodium level, and elevated urine protein level and specific gravity)

• possible hematuria.

Medical treatment

Treatment aims to:

• restore protein balance

• relieve edema
• prevent or control infection
• maintain nutritional status.

Sexually transmitted disease

Children acquire sexually transmitted diseases (STDs) (more than 25 types have been identified) congenitally, during passage through the birth canal, or through voluntary or involuntary sexual contact. (Suspect child molestation in any child under prepubescent age who presents with an STD.)

In most states, adolescents may be treated without parental consent. As a nurse, you'll need to become familiar with the laws in your state and be prepared to offer counseling to adolescents who appear at high risk for STD.

Some of the most common STDs are discussed below:

Gonorrhea. Also known as clap, gonorrhea is caused by a bacterial infection (*Neisseria gonorrhoeae*). Children may acquire the disease directly through sexual contact or in the birth canal. Newborns born with the disease are at risk for ophthalmia neonatorium, scalp abscesses, rhinitis, and pneumonia. Incubation period is 3 to 7 days.

Syphilis. Caused by a bacterial infection (*Treponema pallidum*), syphilis may be acquired by direct sexual contact (95% of all cases), by use of a contaminated needle, or congenitally (the disease may be transmitted to the fetus at any stage during pregnancy). The disease, which has an incubation period of 10 to 90 days, occurs most commonly among those age 15 to 25.

Genital herpes. Herpes simplex virus type II (HSV-II), genital herpes may be acquired congenitally or by direct sexual contact. Incubation period is 7 to 21 days.

Chlamydia. The most common STD, chlamydia (also known as nongonococcal urethritis) is caused by a bacterial infection (*Chlamydia trachomatis*). Occurring most frequently among those age 15 to 25, this disease may be acquired through direct sexual contact or in the birth canal. Frequently, chlamydia and gonorrhea occur together. Infants with this disease are at risk for conjunctivitis, pneumonia, and otitis media. Incubation period is 1 to 3 weeks.

Trichomoniasis. Caused by a flagellated protozoan infection (*Trichomonas vaginalis*), trichomoniasis may be contracted through direct sexual contact or in the vaginal passage during birth. This disease occurs more commonly in heavy smokers.

Candidiasis. Formerly known as moniliasis, candidiasis is caused by a yeast infection (*Candida albicans*). Not necessarily sexually contracted, this disease also can be transmitted by hand contact. Candidiasis occurs commonly during pregnancy and may be transmitted to the neonate during vaginal passage (thrush); it also is common with antibiotic use.

Venereal warts. Caused by a human papilloma virus (HPV) (condylomata acuminata), veneral warts are acquired through direct sexual contact. This disease occurs most commonly among those age 15 to 29.

Assessment
Frequently encountered data for STDs include the following:

Gonorrhea
Boys
• penile discharge and dysuria
• perineal pain
• symptoms of pharyngitis
• burning rectal pain
• blood or mucus in stool
Girls
Although girls may be asymptomatic, the following symptoms may occur:
• frequent urination or dysuria
• vaginal discharge
• symptoms of pharyngitis
• abdominal pain, fever, or vomiting
• arthritis, meningitis, or perihepatic symptoms
• sterility

Syphilis
Boys and girls
• Primary: painless chancre that heals spontaneously in 10 to 90 days
• Secondary: rash and flulike symptoms that disappear in 2 weeks
• Latency period: no symptoms; lasts up to 30 years
• Tertiary: brain damage, paralysis, and heart disease
• Congenital: rhinitis, rash, fever, anemia, jaundice, notched teeth, bone damage, kidney disease, pneumonia, meningitis, and blindness

Genital herpes
Boys and girls
• painful vesicular lesions (may be oral or genital)
• fever, chills, headache, nausea, vomiting, lymphadenopathy, and malaise
• in neonates: high morbidity and mortality associated with congenital herpes

Chlamydia
Boys
• penile discharge
• dysuria

Girls
• abdominal pain
• cervicitis
• salpingitis
• mucopurulent discharge
• burning of vulva

Trichomoniasis
Boys
• usually asymptomatic
Girls
• frothy, greenish-yellow, foul-smelling discharge
• possible pruritus

Candidiasis
Boys
May be asymptomatic or have the following symptoms:
• penile pruritus
• rash
Girls
• white, thick discharge that resembles cottage cheese
• severe pruritus
• vulvar irritation

Veneral warts
Boys
• painless papules on the penis, rectum, or throat (papules bleed easily).
Girls
• painless papules on the vagina, cervix, rectum, or throat (papules bleed easily).
Note: About 91% of all patients with cervical cancer have a history of HPV infection.

Nursing diagnosis
Potential for Infection: Cross-contamination of Self or Other Children related to caring for infected patients
Desired outcome: Infection is confined to the diagnosed individual.

Interventions
1. Institute isolation or infection precautions, as recommended.
2. Observe meticulous hand-washing technique.
3. Teach the child and family about the prevention and spreading of disease.
4. Administer medications promptly to control or destroy responsible organisms.
5. Observe, record, and report the child's response to medications.

Nursing diagnosis

Knowledge Deficit related to lack of information on the transmission, course, and possible long-term effects of STDs

Desired outcome: The caregiver and child (as appropriate) verbalize an understanding of the transmission, course, and possible long-term effects of the disease.

Interventions

1. Build rapport with the adolescent. (Being a student nurse may be an advantage in this situation; the adolescent may find it easier to identify with a student.)
2. Avoid judgmental attitudes.
3. Assess the child's and family's knowledge about STDs, including mode of transmission, signs and symptoms, treatment, prevention, and possible long-term effects.
4. Stress the importance of prenatal care, if appropriate. (Congenital syphilis represents a failure in prenatal care.)
5. Dispel any myths or misconceptions. (Adolescents often believe that birth control pills will protect them against STDs.)
6. Stress the importance of follow-up care.

Medical diagnosis

The medical diagnosis for STDs is based on the following:

Gonorrhea
• modified Thayer Martin culture
• Gram stain (to test for gram-negative diplococcus)

Syphilis
• positive Venereal Disease Research Laboratories (VDRL), rapid plasma reagin (RPR), or plasmacrit (PCT) test
• dark-field examination
• positive fluorescent treponemal antibody-absorption (FTA-ABS) test

Genital herpes
• viral culture
• Papanicolaou (Pap) smear

Chlamydia
• immunoassay
• tissue cell culture

Trichomoniasis
• wet saline mount of vaginal discharge
• Pap smear
• culture of organism

Candidiasis
• saline or potassium hydroxide wet prep
• Pap smear

Venereal warts
• clinical findings
• biopsy (if diagnosis is uncertain)
• aceto-white test.

Medical treatment

Treatment for STD is as follows:

Gonorrhea

Treatment, which is on an outpatient basis unless the child has evidence of pelvic inflammatory disease or disseminated infection, may include:

• administration of penicillin or ampicillin with probenecid (to delay excretion and potentiate action)

• administration of tetracycline or erythromycin if the child is allergic to penicillin

• administration of spectinomycin for resistant cases.

Syphilis

Treatment, which is usually on an outpatient basis unless the patient is an infant or has systemic symptoms, may include:

• administration of penicillin or erythromycin

• administration of tetracycline if the child is allergic to penicillin.

Genital herpes

Treatment includes administration of acyclovir to control the disease only; this medication will not cure the disease.

Chlamydia

Treatment includes:

• administration of tetracycline

• administration of erythromycin if the patient is pregnant.

Trichomoniasis

Treatment includes administration of metronidazole.

Candidiasis

Treatment includes administration of miconazole nitrate 2%, butoconazole nitrate, Mycolog, or nystatin.

Venereal warts

Treatment includes:

• cryosurgery

• electrosurgery

• laser therapy

• administration of podophyllum resin

• administration of fluorouracil

• administration of interferon.

Urinary tract infection

Among the most common disorders affecting children (second only to upper respiratory tract infections), urinary tract infections (UTIs) are classified as either lower or upper infections. Lower UTIs involve the urethra and bladder; upper UTIs affect the ureters and kidneys.

Although viruses, yeasts, and fungi sometimes cause UTIs, the primary pathogens are bacteria (especially *Escherichia coli*). Organisms gain access to the urinary tract through the urethra, the blood, or the lymphatics. Hematologic transmission commonly occurs during the newborn period, affecting both sexes with equal frequency. At all other ages, UTIs occur more frequently among girls.

UTIs can be uncomplicated, complicated, or chronic. Uncomplicated UTIs, characterized as having no associated underlying structural or neurologic lesions, usually respond well to drug therapy. Occurring most commonly among children age 2 to 6 and sexually active adolescents, uncomplicated UTIs usually are treated on an outpatient basis.

Complicated UTIs are associated with repeated infections that produce inflammatory changes or with obstruction of urine drainage by structural or neurologic disorders. Acutely ill children, such as those with symptoms of septic shock, and children requiring correction of structural defects usually are hospitalized.

Chronic UTIs may result in destruction of kidney tissue, anemia, hypertension, failure to grow and develop, and eventual renal failure.

Assessment

Wide variations in signs and symptoms have been reported with UTIs. Frequently encountered data include the following:

Subjective
- frequency
- urgency
- dysuria (manifested in infancy by screaming during voiding)
- nocturia
- chronic constipation
- suprapubic discomfort
- low back pain
- hematuria
- chills and fever
- nausea and vomiting
- perineal pruritus

Objective
- fever of up to 104° F. (40° C.)
- suprapubic tenderness (noted during the examination)
- pallor
- costovertebral angle tenderness (evident during percussion)
- diaper rash or vulvovaginitis
- anemia, hypertension, and failure to thrive (associated with chronic UTIs).

When taking the history, inquire about the use of bubble baths or feminine sprays. Question hygienic practices (such as the direction of wiping and the frequency of underwear changes), and ask about symptoms suggesting pinworm infestation.

Nursing diagnosis

Altered Urinary Elimination Pattern related to inflammation or infection
Desired outcome: The child establishes a normal pattern of elimination.

Interventions

1. Collect or assist with the collection and handling of urine specimens for identification of causative organisms. (This may require a clean-catch midstream urine specimen, placement of a plastic collection bag, catheterization, or suprapubic aspiration.)
2. Monitor the child's intake and output.
3. Observe the character of the child's urine.
4. Administer antibiotics or urinary antiseptics, as ordered, after obtaining cultures.
5. Encourage fluids to prevent crystalluria, especially if the child is taking sulfonamides.
6. Provide an acid-ash diet, unless contraindicated.
7. Prepare the child and caregivers for diagnostic procedures to discover structural anomalies.
8. Provide preoperative and postoperative care of the child requiring corrective surgery (see Section 4).
9. Pay special attention to maintaining patency and preventing complications when urinary drainage tubes are used.

Nursing diagnosis

Potential for Infection: Extension or Introduction of New Organisms related to ineffective treatment or adverse effects of antibiotics
Desired outcome: The UTI is arrested, no additional organisms are introduced, and no adverse reactions to antibiotics develop.

Interventions

1. Monitor the child for signs and symptoms of septicemia.
2. Use careful aseptic technique.
3. Administer antibiotics or urinary antiseptics, as ordered.
4. Observe, record, and report responses to medications.
5. Monitor the child for signs and symptoms of candidiasis, a common adverse effect of antibiotic therapy; observe for vulvovaginitis, pruritus, irritation, or discharge from the vagina; and inspect the oral cavity for thrush.
6. Carefully cleanse and dry the perineum after the child voids or has a bowel movement.
7. Practice and instruct the family on careful hand-washing techniques.

Nursing diagnosis

Altered Comfort: Dyspnea, Flank Pain, or Abdominal Discomfort related to inflammation or infection of the urinary tract
Desired outcome: The child verbalizes relief of discomfort.

Interventions

1. Encourage fluids, as permitted and tolerated, to dilute urine.
2. Apply local heat (such as a heating pad or sitz bath), as ordered.
3. Administer urinary analgesics, such as phenazopyridine hydrochloride, if ordered; prepare the child and caregivers for urine discoloration associated with this medication.

Nursing diagnosis

Knowledge Deficit related to postdischarge management of the child
Desired outcome: The caregiver or child (as appropriate) verbalizes an understanding of discharge planning to bring about and maintain full recovery.

Interventions

1. Include the following information in discharge instructions:
• Avoid giving the child tub baths (especially bubble baths or baths with water softeners).
• Make sure the child wears loose-fitting white cotton underwear.
• Check for pinworms if the child is seen scratching. (Pinworm infection occurs frequently among children who thumbsuck or bite fingernails).
• Make sure the child's perineum is wiped from front to back.
• Avoid overdistention of the bladder. (The child may have to be called in from play and reminded to void.)
• Acidify the child's urine with an acid-ash diet, if not contraindicated. (Refer the caregiver to the hospital dietitian.)
• Make sure the child is adequately hydrated.
• Take measures to prevent constipation; mechanical obstruction of urine could result.
• Report signs and symptoms of UTI.
• Use nitrite or glucose indicator strip tests to test the child's urine at home.
• Make sure the child receives all medications and complies with the full regimen, even if symptoms have subsided.
• Keep all follow-up appointments.

Medical diagnosis

The medical diagnosis for UTI is based on:
• urine sample showing more than 100,000 bacterial colonies/ml
• urinalysis showing cloudy, malodorous urine with white blood cells, casts, protein, red blood cells, and pus
• complete blood count (to check for leukocytosis).
   Further studies are recommended after the first UTI in boys and after the second UTI in girls, including:
• intravenous pyelography
• cystoscopy
• voiding cystourethrography.

Medical treatment

Treatment aims to eliminate the responsible organisms, diagnose and correct obstructive structural anomalies, and provide education to decrease the risk of future infections. The child with a history of UTI will require annual follow-up evaluations.

Wilms' tumor (nephroblastoma)

A nephroblastoma of the kidney, Wilms' tumor usually occurs in infants and toddlers. Children diagnosed before age 1 have the most favorable prognosis for cure because the tumor is more likely to be encapsulated without metastasis.

Usually unilateral (90%), Wilms' tumor grows rapidly and metastasizes early, most frequently to the lungs and possibly extending to regional lymph nodes or, through the renal vein, to the inferior vena cava. Anomalies associated with this tumor include genitourinary deformities, malformation of the external ear, microcephaly, and aniridia (absence of the iris). Some research supports the possibility of genetic transmission.

Histologically, Wilms' tumor is classified as either favorable or unfavorable. Five stages of involvement have been established as criteria for determining treatment protocols. These stages progress from I (with unilateral involvement and no metastasis) to stage V (with bilateral kidney involvement and metastasis to the liver, lung, brain, and bone).

Assessment

Frequently encountered data for Wilms' tumor include the following:

Subjective

• a lump in the belly (reported by the caregiver)
• occasional fever
• abdominal pain
• vomiting, malaise, anorexia, and weight loss (later in disease's course)

Objective

• firm, nontender, palpable mass (usually left-sided)
• fever
• hypertension (occasionally)
• hematuria (occasionally)
• cachexia, anemia, and respiratory distress (later in disease's course).

Nursing diagnosis (pre-treatment)

Potential for Injury: Rupture of the Tumor Capsule and Spread of Malignant Cells related to palpation of the abdomen
Desired outcome: Handling of tumor mass is avoided to prevent liberation of malignant cells.

Interventions
1. Do *not* palpate the mass.
2. Post a sign over the child's bed stating "Do not palpate my abdomen."
3. Use extreme caution in bathing and handling the child.
4. Accompany the child to and from X-ray sessions and surgery to supervise handling.

Nursing diagnosis (post-treatment)

Potential for Infection (Incisional, Skin, or Respiratory) related to increased susceptibility secondary to radiation or chemotherapy
Desired outcome: The child has no evidence of infection.

Interventions
1. Maintain strict aseptic technique.
2. Prevent contact with infected persons.
3. Provide meticulous skin care, keeping the skin dry and clean.
4. Have the child turn, cough, and deep-breathe to maintain respiratory function.

Nursing diagnosis

Ineffective Individual and Family Coping related to lack of adequate time to prepare for life-threatening illness
Desired outcome: The caregivers and child (as appropriate) demonstrate comfort in making decisions and verbalize adjustment to the diagnosis.

Interventions
1. Clarify the doctor's explanations of tests and procedures for the child and family.
2. Use the limited preoperative time (normally, 24 to 48 hours from admission to surgery) to best advantage by supporting and assisting the family.
3. Consider the nature of the crisis and its potential overwhelming effect on the family in all contacts with them. Comfort them and attempt to ease their confusion.

Nursing diagnosis

Altered Bowel Elimination: Constipation related to effects of post-treatment intestinal edema or failure of peristalsis
Desired outcome: The child has no evidence of intestinal obstruction through the postoperative period and during antimetabolite therapy.

Interventions
1. Monitor the child for signs and symptoms of intestinal obstruction by:
• frequently assessing bowel sounds
• observing, recording, and reporting any vomiting, pain, or distention
• checking for bowel movement.

2. Maintain the patency and function of the nasogastric tube, if applicable.

Nursing diagnosis

Fluid Volume Excess related to effects of inadequate kidney function

Desired outcome: The child's fluid balance is maintained.

Interventions

1. Monitor the child's intake and output to evaluate the function of remaining kidney tissue.
2. Observe, record, and report diminished output.
3. Maintain I.V. therapy at the prescribed rate.

Nursing diagnosis

Knowledge Deficit related to home management of long-term chemotherapy

Desired outcome: The caregivers and child (as appropriate) verbalize an understanding of the need for and the implications of long-term chemotherapy.

Interventions

1. Provide information on the adverse effects of chemotherapy.
2. Suggest ways for managing alopecia, nausea, and other problems.
3. Establish an information source for ready accessibility after discharge.
4. Encourage the child's return to school or other activities and usual discipline practices to maintain as much normalcy as possible.
5. Arrange and stress the importance of follow-up evaluations.

Medical diagnosis

The medical diagnosis for Wilms' tumor is based on:
• computed tomography scan (to elaborate the tumor's location and dimensions)
• intravenous pyelography (to demonstrate distortion of the kidney pelvis and determine if the condition is bilateral)
• venacavogram (to rule out metastasis to the vena cava)
• X-rays of lungs, liver, and skeleton (to rule out metastasis)
• urinalysis
• complete blood count (may show polycythemia from increased erythropoietic activity by tumor cells or evidence of anemia caused by intraabdominal hemorrhage)
• liver function tests (to assess metastatic damage and the ability to metabolize therapeutic drugs).

Medical treatment

The treatment plan is determined by assessing the stage and histologic classification. Surgery is scheduled as soon as possible after diagnosis is made.

Stage I with a favorable histology requires only radical nephrectomy. Other stages are managed with combinations of surgery, radiation, and chemotherapy. Agents usually used include dactinomycin, vincristine, cyclophosphamide, and doxorubicin hydrochloride.

☐ Integumentary and immunologic systems

Children are rarely hospitalized for primary diagnoses of diseases or disorders affecting the skin. However, secondary diagnoses frequently include pathologic changes affecting this complex structure, the body's largest organ.

The intact, tough outer layer of skin acts as a mechanical barrier against invading microorganisms and protects against the loss of essential body constituents. Skin lesions may be caused by various extrinsic agents or may be an intrinsic manifestation of a systemic disorder.

Although the immune system is complex, it may be described simply as the mechanism by which the body recognizes "self" from "nonself." (A foreign substance or antigen stimulates a nonspecific or specific immune defense that attempts to eliminate the nonself.) Immunologic disorders often are life-threatening.

Admission assessment

During the admission assessment, you'll need to take a detailed nursing history and perform a physical examination.

Patient history. Find out about the following:
• Pruritus, pain, and rashes: Does the child have a history of any of these symptoms?
• Hair: Has he experienced any recent hair loss or unusual growth (hirsutism)? Has he noticed a change in the color or texture of his hair? What specific hair products does he use?
• Skin: Has there been a change in the child's usual skin color, texture, or turgor? Has he noticed any changes in existing skin lesions? Does he have any new lesions? How well does his skin usually respond to injury? What types of skin products does he use?
• Nails: Have there been any changes in nail color, shape, markings, or texture? What type of nail products (if any) does he use?
• Sun exposure: How often is the child exposed to the sun? What precautions (if any) does he take for such exposure?
• Chemical exposure: Is the child exposed to any chemicals, including cleaning compounds, medications, and craft materials?
• Allergies: Is there a seasonal pattern to any of the child's symptoms?
• Stress: Is there any relationship betwen the child's symptoms and stress?
• Infections: How frequently does the child have infections?

Family history. Ask whether there is a family history of allergy with skin manifestations. Also ask about a history of skin cancer, congenital skin lesions, bleeding tendencies or anemia, joint diseases, and early death of a family member from overwhelming infection.

Physical assessment

Examine the child's lesions carefully, noting their distinctive characteristics to help determine the pathologic process. Use adequate natural or artificial light, such as a Wood's (fluorescent) light (helpful for viewing abnormal pigmentation). A low-powered magnifying lens also may be useful.

Determine whether the lesions are primary or secondary. Primary lesions refer to skin changes produced by the causative factor; secondary lesions refer to changes of the primary lesions produced by rubbing, scratching, treatment, or healing.

Describe the lesions in terms of the following information (see *Glossary of integumentary terms* for common terms and their definitions):
• distribution pattern (any lesions associated with a specific area)
• specific body areas affected
• size, shape, and arrangement (such as grouped, ringed, or linear)
• symptoms (such as the type and intensity of pruritus)
• sensory changes (such as pain, burning, crawling sensation, sensitivity, or diminished feeling)
• factors that aggravate symptoms.

Acne vulgaris

A disorder of the sebaceous glands related to oversecretion of sebum, acne affects almost all adolescents to a certain degree. Lesions include two basic types: comedones (blackheads or whiteheads) and inflamed lesions (infected cysts that lead to scarring). Multiple factors, including androgen production, heredity, emotional stress, the premenstrual period, and (in some cases) food items, appear to contribute to the severity of the condition.

Although not a cause for hospitalization, acne may affect the hospitalized preadolescent or adolescent patient; nurses may need to assume routine management of the condition while the patient is hospitalized.

Assessment

Acne appears as lesions on the face, neck, shoulders, or upper trunk; it may consist of noninflamed comedones (whiteheads or blackheads) or inflamed lesions (papules, pustules, or cysts).

During the patient history, ask about possible causative factors, such as premenstrual period, ingestion of steroids or other drugs, occupational environment, heredity, and food (rarely a factor).

GLOSSARY OF INTEGUMENTARY TERMS

Abrasion—scraping away of a portion of skin or mucous membrane by mechanical means

Bulla—fluid-filled vesicle greater than 1 cm; large vesicle or bleb (for example, second-degree burn or impetigo)

Crust—temporary covering of a lesion from dried blood or serum

Ecchymosis—black and blue mark

Erythema—reddened area

Excoriation—destruction of the epidermis from chemicals, burns, or other trauma

Macule—flat spot, less than 1 cm in diameter, with color alteration (for example, a freckle or measles)

Papule—small, solid elevation of skin (less than 1 cm) (for example, a wart or an early pimple)

Petechiae—pinpoint, tiny hemorrhages in superficial layers of the epidermis

Pustule—vesicle filled with pus (usually staphylococcal or streptococcal) (for example, acne or impetigo)

Vesicle—small, superficial elevation of skin (less than 1 cm) containing serous or blood-tinged fluid (for example, chicken pox, poison ivy, or a blister)

Wheal—round or flat-topped, irregular shape resulting from edema in the upper dermis (for example, mosquito bites or urticaria)

Nursing diagnosis
Impaired Skin Integrity related to inflammation and infection of lesions
Desired outcome: The child remains free of inflamed lesions that lead to infected cysts and scarring.

Interventions
1. Elicit information from the child or caregivers concerning the routine care before illness.
2. Obtain cleansing agents, astringents, or topical preparations, as ordered.
3. Assist with or implement treatment.
4. Monitor the status of lesions to minimize the risk of infection.
5. Acknowledge and discuss the condition as a temporary state.
6. Avoid embarrassing the child about his condition; use humor judiciously.

Nursing diagnosis
Disturbance in Self-concept: Altered Body Image related to change in appearance secondary to skin lesions and scarring
Desired outcome: The patient uses skin management techniques to minimize the number and severity of lesions.

Interventions
1. Explain the cause of the condition as related to factors of hormonal imbalance and heredity.
2. Emphasize the rationale for skin cleansing procedures.
3. Encourage the integration of good health practices into the child's daily routine (such as daily bathing, frequent or daily shampoos, exercise, and adequate sleep).
4. Discuss dietary factors. (Although rarely a causative factor, certain foods may be identified as the problem; affirm the need to eliminate them from the diet.)

5. Assist in identifying ways to camouflage lesions.
6. Affirm the normalcy of the process as a stage in human development.

Medical diagnosis
The medical diagnosis for acne vulgaris is based on:
• inspection of lesions
• history of exacerbations (degree of condition varies; usually self-limited, but may result in a disturbed self-image and lifelong scarring).

Medical treatment
Treatment focuses on the child's overall health status, emphasizing the need for a well-balanced diet, exercise, and rest. Specific treatments for acne types include the following:
Noninflammatory acne
• use of cleansing soaps, astringents, peeling and drying techniques, lotions and creams, and tretinoin cream or lotion
• professional removal of comedones
Inflammatory acne
• use of tetracyline or erythromycin systemically
• incision and drainage of cysts
• dermabrasion
• use of isotretinoin systemically (may cause birth defects and damage blood cell formation).

Acquired immunodeficiency syndrome (AIDS)
Children of parents with AIDS or AIDS-related complex (ARC) are at risk for this deadly disease. Human immunodeficiency virus (HIV), the causative agent responsible for AIDS, alters T4 cells and the T4 receptors of other cells, resulting in blockage of the cellular immune response. The virus, which spreads throughout the body on macrophage cells, attacks all body systems; the central nervous system (CNS) is especially vulnerable.

T cells normally function to protect the body against most viral, fungal, protozoan, and slow-growing bacterial infections and possibly initiate a cell-mediated immune response to malignant cells. T cell dysfunction, which occurs in AIDS, has life-threatening implications for those affected with the disease.

Studies suggest that transplacental transmission of the virus occurs in more than 50% of pregnancies in which the mother is infected. If the mother is infected with the virus, breast-feeding is contraindicated.

Children diagnosed as having AIDS have a less than favorable prognosis if onset of symptoms begins before age 1 rather than age 2 to 3. Children who received blood transfusions before 1984, especially hemophiliacs, are at high risk.

A confirmed diagnosis is difficult during the first 15 months because of the presence of maternal antibody. A negative culture or antigen may not be interpreted to indicate that the child is free from the infection.

A provisional diagnosis may be based on the presence of an underlying cellular immunodeficiency-related disease as evidenced by such symptoms as diarrhea (possibly of an unknown etiology) and lymphocytic interstitial pneumonia. Later, the diagnosis may be confirmed using the Western Blot test or the enzyme-linked immunosorbent assay (ELISA). Usually, the ELISA is used first, although it has a high rate of false-positive results. The Western Blot test is used for confirmation.

Assessment
Frequently encountered data for AIDS include the following:

Subjective
• high-risk parent (may be bisexual, sexually promiscuous, an I.V. drug user, a hemophiliac, or a blood transfusion recipient)
• hemophilia
• development of the following symptoms (initially, child is a healthy infant):
    —intermittent episodes of diarrhea
    —repeated respiratory infections
    —inability to tolerate feedings

Objective
• failure to thrive
• persistent diarrhea (cryptosporidiosis or unknown etiology)
• lymphadenopathy
• acute respiratory infection
• fever and tachypnea
• respiratory distress
• oral candidal infection (white patches)
• salivary gland enlargement
• hepatosplenomegaly.

Nursing diagnosis
Potential for Infection related to decreased resistance associated with immunodeficiency and malnutrition
Desired outcome: The child remains free of additional infection as evidenced by no signs or symptoms of infection and an improved general physical condition (weight gain, improved feeding, and increased strength and activity tolerance).

Interventions
1. Monitor the child for the following:
• signs and symptoms of additional infection
• increased temperature and pulse and respiratory rates
• symptoms of respiratory distress, including dyspnea, cyanosis, and retractions

• redness, swelling, or drainage of skin areas
• positive cultures (urine, stool, or other body fluids).
2. Institute isolation protocol, including strict hand-washing technique and use of a gown and gloves when in direct contact with the child (see *AIDS precautions*).
3. Restrict personnel with potential communicable disease, such as skin and upper respiratory tract infections.
4. Maintain meticulous aseptic technique when caring for any invasive tubes (such as I.V. lines, catheters, endotracheal tubes, and nasogastric tubes) and related body sites.
5. Keep the child's environment clean.

Nursing diagnosis

Altered Nutrition: Less Than Body Requirements related to decreased oral intake secondary to inability to tolerate feedings, malaise and fatigue, persistent diarrhea, or increased metabolism associated with infection (specify)
Desired outcome: The child returns to an adequate nutritional status as evidenced by progress in growth and development.

Interventions

1. Assess and monitor the child's nutritional status on a regular basis, using growth charts, developmental screening tests, and blood chemistry studies.
2. Take necessary measures to correct the child's failure to thrive (see "Failure to thrive" in Section 3).
3. Provide care for oral lesions by gently cleaning mucous membranes and applying medication, as ordered.
4. Apply a topical anesthetic agent (such as Xylocaine Viscous), as ordered, before feedings.

Medical diagnosis

The medical diagnosis for AIDS is based on:
• the patient history
• evidence of failure to thrive
• workup for immunodeficiency
• neutropenia, thrombocytopenia, hemolytic anemia, decrease in total number of T cells and helper T cells, alteration in the T4:T8 ratio
• diseases indicative of underlying cellular immunodeficiency, including:
    —*Pneumocystis carinii* pneumonia
    —frequent routine bacterial infections
    —candidiasis
    —cytomegalovirus (occurring after age 1 month and causing pulmonary, GI tract, or disseminated infection)
    —HIV (positive antigen noted after age 15 months).

AIDS PRECAUTIONS

Institute the following precautions when caring for a child with AIDS.

Precautions	Comments
Private room	Keeping the patient in a private room is necessary for the child's protection as well as for the protection of others.
Gown and gloves	Wear a gown and gloves when in direct contact with the patient or with blood and body fluids.
Hand washing	Wash hands upon entering and leaving the patient's room and immediately after contacting blood or body fluids. (Wash gloved hands.)
Mask	Wear a mask during sustained contact with a coughing patient, while suctioning respiratory secretions, or when blood may contaminate mucous membranes.
Needles and syringes	Never recap or clip needles or syringes. Always place them in a puncture-proof container.
Specimens	Place a biohazard warning on all specimens.
Food service materials	Use disposable cups, plates, and utensils for all of the patient's meals.
Asepsis	Make sure that all surfaces are clean; sterilize all of the patient's linens.

Medical treatment

Initial treatment includes:
• therapy for the child's specific disease state (steroids effective in lymphocytic interstitial pneumonia)
• protective isolation to prevent nosocomial infections
• nutritional support.
   After diagnosis, treatment includes:
• administration of prophylactic antibiotics
• blood and stool cultures to identify potential life-threatening infections
• administration of steroids and I.V. immune globulin during acute episodes of infection
• annual cranial computed tomography scans to detect CNS deterioration.

Atopic dermatitis (infantile eczema)

An antigen-antibody disorder also known as infantile eczema when it affects young children, atopic dermatitis results from allergy. The allergen may be ingested, inhaled, or transmitted by direct skin contact.

Atopic dermatitis produces skin lesions that begin as red, scaling areas (usually on the head, neck, and flexor surfaces) and progress to small vesicles that break and weep, forming crusts. Itching may be intense.

Assessment

Frequently encountered data for atopic dermatitis include:

Subjective
• irritability or inability to rest or sleep
• itching (as evidenced by attempts to scratch)

Objective
• lesions (erythematous and edematous)
• unaffected skin areas that become dry and rough
• lymphadenopathy proximal to lesions
• secondary infection (pustules).

Nursing diagnosis

Altered Comfort related to presence of skin lesions
Desired outcome: The child verbalizes comfort.

Interventions
1. Assist the child and caregivers in identifying and eliminating allergens.
2. Protect the child against invading microorganisms (protective isolation).
3. Minimize damage from scratching by trimming the child's nails; also, have the child wear gloves and cotton clothing with long sleeves and legs (as necessary).
4. Cleanse the diaper area frequently with plain water.
5. Promote good health by scheduling the child's meals at a time when he is rested and using comfort measures that encourage rest or sleep periods.
6. Administer therapeutic soaks or tub baths with cornstarch preparations, oatmeal (Aveeno) preparations, or bicarbonate of soda; make sure the water temperature is tepid.
7. Use clothing and linen that has been thoroughly cleansed and rinsed.
8. Monitor the status of the lesions to evaluate the effectiveness of treatment.
9. Avoid exposing the child to lanolin, wool products, and feather pillows or mattresses.

Nursing diagnosis

Altered Comfort related to pruritus
Desired outcome: The child expresses relief of dry skin as evidenced by verbalization, less scratching and rubbing of skin, and less irritability, which result in improved eating and sleeping.

Interventions
1. Administer topical or systemic medications to control pruritus.
2. Administer sedatives and antibiotics, as ordered.
3. Provide emotional support to caregivers (irritability related to the disorder may be exhausting for the caregivers).

Medical diagnosis
The medical diagnosis for atopic dermatitis is based on identification of the causative allergen by:
• taking a careful history
• use of an elimination diet
• controlling the home environment.

Medical treatment
Treatment may include:
• removal of allergen by feeding the child a hypoallergenic diet and removing the allergen from the child's home
• avoiding the use of soap and hot water
• using cleansing and lubricating solutions, antiseptic soaks, wet soaks, or dressings
• administering topical steroids
• administering medication to control pruritus, including antihistamines (such as diphenhydramine), sedatives (such as chloral hydrate), and antipruritics (such as hydroxyzine)
• administering systemic antibiotics for infections.

Diaper dermatitis
Commonly known as diaper rash, diaper dermatitis causes skin eruptions or inflammation from frequent and prolonged contact with urine, feces, soaps, or chemicals in the diaper area. If the involved skin area is in direct contact with the diaper itself, irritating chemicals are usually the cause.

Seborrheic dermatitis, an inflammatory process also associated with the diaper area, usually manifests in the areas around the groin and gluteal folds. Loss of skin integrity could lead to invasion of organisms, causing impetigo or candidiasis.

Assessment
Frequently encountered data for diaper dermatitis include:
• lesions and inflammation in the diaper area. Observing the lesions and areas involved may indicate the cause:
   —Lesions on the buttocks, inner thigh, scrotum, and mons pubis are usually caused by detergents, soaps, ammonia, and fecal waste.
   —Lesions on surfaces touching the diaper, such as the groin and gluteal folds, are caused by intertrigo or seborrhea; they may become infected with candidiasis, especially if maternal vaginal candidiasis exists.

• vesicles or bullae (indicate impetigo)
• beet-red lesions with accompanying satellite lesions (indicate candidal infection).

Nursing diagnosis

Potential for Infection related to prolonged skin contact with urine, feces, or other chemical agents
Desired outcome: The child has no evidence of infection.

Interventions

1. Remove occlusive diaper coverings to permit evaporation.
2. Change the child's diaper as soon as it becomes wet.
3. Cleanse the perineal area with each soiling; keep in mind the following information:
• Wipe the area with a wet cloth to remove urine.
• Avoid disposable wet towels; agents in the towel may cause a sensitivity reaction.
• Thoroughly cleanse the area after each stool; diarrhea may necessitate immersing the area in a tub filled with tepid water.
4. Allow the area to dry thoroughly. (If necessary, cautiously use a hair blower on a low heat setting.)
5. Avoid using talcum powder because the child may aspirate the powder, causing lung problems. (*Note:* Cornstarch is a culture medium for *Candida,* and baking soda may cause metabolic acidosis.)
6. Avoid applying an occlusive ointment to the inflamed area.
7. Use soft, thoroughly laundered, and sterile diapers (commercially laundered diapers are preferred). (Instruct caregivers to soak diapers in Diaperene, wash them in hot water with a mild laundry soap, and rinse them twice.)
8. If disposable diapers are used, choose a type that allows some evaporation, as some contain irritating agents.
9. Teach the caregivers ways to prevent diaper rash and appropriate interventions for early reversal of its onset.

Medical diagnosis

The medical diagnosis for diaper dermatitis is based on:
• inspection
• culture and sensitivity of secretions.

Medical treatment

Treatment includes:
• application of a topical glucocorticoid (1% hydrocortisone cream)
• use of anticandidal dusting powder or cream.

Impetigo

A highly contagious skin infection in young infants, impetigo is caused by staphylococcus or streptococcus bacteria. Lesions typically begin as reddish macules that become vesicular and eventually rupture, forming thick, yellow-red, peripherally spreading crusts.

Impetigo occurs most commonly among malnourished children who live in overcrowded, unsanitary environments. The extent of involvement may be minimal to extensive, requiring hospitalization. Although older children are less threatened by the condition, infants may be seriously affected. Hospitalized children are isolated on the pediatric unit.

Assessment

Frequently encountered data for impetigo include the following:
• reddish macules that become vesicular, rupturing easily and leaving a superficial moist erosion; exudate dries to form a heavy, honey-colored crust
• peripherally spreading lesions with irregular but well-defined outlines
• pruritus.

Nursing diagnosis

Impaired Skin Integrity related to the effects of scratching associated with pruritus
Desired outcome: The child has improved skin integrity as demonstrated by the healing of existing lesions, no evidence of lesion extension, and less scratching.

Interventions

1. Institute protective (reverse) and wound and skin isolation techniques, including use of gowns, gloves, and aseptic technique when treating lesions.
2. Trim the child's nails.
3. Clothe the child in long-sleeved cotton shirts and long cotton pants.
4. Cleanse lesions to remove crusts before applying topical antibiotics.
5. Administer systemic and local antibiotics and observe for adverse effects.
6. Administer antihistamines or antipruritics to reduce pruritus during the acute phase.

Medical diagnosis

The medical diagnosis for impetigo is based on:
• inspection of lesions
• culture and sensitivity of exudate.

Medical treatment

Treatment includes:
• careful cleaning and removal of crusts
• topical application of bactericidal ointment
• systemic administration (oral) of penicillin or erythromycin
• administration of medications for pruritus.

Kawasaki disease (mucocutaneous lymph node syndrome [MLNS])

An acute, febrile systemic disorder that occurs primarily in infants and young children, Kawasaki disease has the highest incidence in Japan and other Oriental countries. Recently, incidence of the disease has increased in the United States.

Although the exact cause of Kawasaki disease is unknown, certain epidemiologic evidence suggests an infectious etiology; however, serology and culture of body fluids have not identified a causative organism. Research suggests the possibility of a retrovirus because of the transient impairment of the immunologic regulatory system (T4, T8, and B cells) associated with the disease.

Kawasaki disease principally attacks the cardiovascular system. (Morbidity in the heart or one of its vessels is about 20%.) Usually, death occurs from coronary thrombosis (within 28 to 31 days after onset), stenosis of the coronary artery (after 40 days), and aneurysm ("string of pearls" effect). Improved treatment, however, has resulted in a decreasing mortality.

Assessment

Frequently encountered data for Kawasaki disease include the following:

Acute febrile phase (lasting 1 to 14 days)

Subjective
• high fever
• red, dry lips
• red, swollen hands and feet
• irritability
• diarrhea and earache (sometimes)
• photosensitivity

Objective
• spiking fever lasting 5 days (unresponsive to antibiotics)
• oropharyngeal erythema ("strawberry tongue")
• infected conjunctiva
• edema with induration of the hands and feet
• erythema of the palms and soles
• erythematous rash
• cervical lymphadenopathy

Subacute phase (lasting 10 to 25 days)

Subjective
• joint pain
• irritability
• decreased appetite

Objective
• desquamation of the palms and soles
• arthritis
• no fever

Convalescent phase (lasting 25 days or more)
Subjective
• well feeling
• Beau's lines (on fingers and toes).

Nursing diagnosis
Hyperthermia (Severe, Spiking, Unresponsive to Antibiotics) related to the effects of early (acute) phase of Kawasaki disease
Desired outcome: The child has a controlled temperature and no evidence of seizures, dehydration, or neurologic or other complications.

Interventions
1. Be especially alert to clinical findings, such as the characteristic spiking 5-day fever pattern (which is unresponsive to antibiotics) associated with this disease; early treatment has been effective in preventing long-term complications.
2. Take the following measures to control fever:
• Administer aspirin; 80 to 150 mg/kg/day may be ordered during the acute phase. Note the following information:
  —Never give aspirin on an empty stomach.
  —Observe the child for adverse reactions, including tinnitus, epigastric distress (nausea, vomiting, and heartburn), GI bleeding, hematuria, and acidosis with hyperventilation.
• Give tepid sponge baths.
• Regulate the environmental temperature to remain between 68° and 70° F. (20° and 21° C.).
• Provide adequate hydration; this may require the administration of I.V. fluids.

Nursing diagnosis
Fluid Volume Deficit related to increased metabolism secondary to elevated temperature
Desired outcome: The child maintains fluid balance.

Interventions
1. Control the child's fever by using the measures outlined above.
2. Monitor for signs and symptoms of dehydration and electrolyte imbalance by:
• accurately measuring intake and output
• taking and recording daily weights
• assessing skin turgor and mucous membranes
• measuring vital signs frequently
• reviewing laboratory reports (hemoglobin, hematocrit, and electrolyte levels).

Nursing diagnosis
Altered Cardiac Output, Decreased: Hemodynamic Problems re-

lated to thrombotic episodes and aneurysms of coronary arteries
Desired outcome: The child has no cardiac complications and experiences complete recovery.

Interventions
1. Assist with observing and reporting clinical findings; therapy to prevent coronary artery disease is effective if given within 10 days of onset.
2. Administer I.V. immune globulin (the latest therapy), as ordered.
3. Encourage compliance with maintenance therapy, which may include:
• administering aspirin 3 to 5 mg/kg/day on a long-term basis
• administering dipyridamole (often prescribed with aspirin)
• follow-up visits for EKGs and platelet counts. (Intense supervision is critical.)
4. Teach the caregivers the signs and symptoms of aspirin toxicity and which adverse reactions to report to the doctor.

Medical diagnosis
The medical diagnosis for Kawasaki disease is based on:
• spiking fever lasting 5 days as well as at least four of the following signs and symptoms:
   —bilateral injected bulbar conjunctiva
   —red, cracked lips and oral mucous membranes
   —edema and erythema of the hands and feet with desquamation of the palms and soles
   —erythematous rash
   —cervical lymphadenopathy
• laboratory findings, including:
   —leukocytosis (20,000/mm^3 or more with elevated neutrophil count)
   —sedimentation rate greater than 50%
   —elevated C-reactive protein levels
   —elevated platelet count (600,000 to 2,000,000/mm^3 platelets; after the acute phase)
   —moderate anemia
   —EKG changes
   —abnormal echocardiograph studies.
(*Note:* Although no specific laboratory test confirms the disease, some studies are used to complete the clinical diagnosis.)

Medical treatment
Treatment aims to control fever, prevent dehydration and electrolyte imbalance, and prevent cardiac morbidity or mortality by use of I.V. immune globulin, aspirin, and persantine. Long-term follow-up is essential.

Sepsis

Also known as bacteremia or septicemia, sepsis is the wide-spread distribution of a bacterial infection through the blood-stream. The diminished immune response of infants and young children places this age-group at particular risk. Neonatal sepsis occurs most commonly in premature infants and those born after a traumatic labor or delivery. Before the use of antibiotics in treating sepsis, mortality approached 90%.

Bacterial invasion may occur through the skin, mucous membranes (nose, pharynx, ears, or eyes), or internal systems (GI, respiratory, urinary, or nervous). Because of a poor anti-inflammatory reaction at the invasion site, the patient may have a lack of symptoms at the specific infection site.

Assessment

Frequently encountered data for sepsis include the following:

Subjective
• lack of desired response to treatment of a known infection
• complaints of the child's "not doing well" or "not looking right"
• poor appetite
• diminished activity

Objective
• fever (often intermittent with wide diurnal variations, possibly spiking)
• chills and cold, clammy skin
• circulatory changes (dysrhythmias or tachycardia)
• respiratory changes (irregular, with periods of apnea, tachypnea, dyspnea, and retractions)
• irritability
• petechial or purpural skin lesions.

Nursing diagnosis

Altered Cardiac Output, Decreased: Sustained Tachycardia related to increased metabolic demand associated with fever
Desired outcome: The child's heart rate remains within a normal range.

Interventions
1. Take appropriate measures to decrease the child's physiologic stress.
2. Institute bed rest with limited activity.
3. Administer high-potency nutrients in easily consumed and digested foods. (Parenteral nutrition may be ordered.)
4. Decrease environmental stress.
5. Keep the child's room temperature cool; make sure the air is well circulated.
6. Limit stimuli from other patients and visitors other than the primary caregivers.

7. Maximize sleep and rest periods by scheduling assessment and procedures.

8. Provide psychological support; maintain a calm attitude.

Nursing diagnosis

Hyperthermia related to increased metabolic rate resulting from bacteremia

Desired outcome: The body response to bacterial infection resolves as evidenced by a normal body temperature.

Interventions

1. Monitor and assess vital signs frequently (may include central venous pressure).

2. Assess the child's neurologic response. (Meningitis may be a sequela of sepsis in young children.)

3. Monitor laboratory studies, especially coagulation studies. (Septic shock may result in disseminated intravascular coagulation.)

4. Administer antipyretics, such as acetaminophen, as ordered.

5. To promote surface cooling, dress the child in light clothing and remove blankets. (Heat loss from the body occurs by radiation, conduction, and convection.)

6. Cool the child's environment by using fans.

7. Administer tepid sponge baths, as ordered.

8. Administer oxygen, as ordered.

9. Provide and regulate a hypothermia blanket, as ordered.

10. Administer I.V. fluids and electrolytes, as ordered, to maintain hydration and electrolyte balance.

11. Administer antibiotics, as ordered.

Medical diagnosis

The medical diagnosis for sepsis is based on:

• signs and symptoms

• identification of the causative organism through:
  —analysis of the potential primary source of infection (for example, specimens from the naso-oro-pharyngeal cavity, urine, stool, or cerebrospinal fluid)
  —blood culture (collect the specimen during or immediately after a fever "spike"; usually collected on three separate occasions).

Medical treatment

Diagnosis may not be definitive before instituting antibiotic therapy. Treatment includes administration of broad-spectrum I.V. antibiotics for a minimum of 10 days.

Supportive therapy includes maintaining fluid and electrolyte balance, providing nutritional needs (may be parenteral; the oral route may be discontinued temporarily in infants), and maintaining thermal regulation.

Severe combined immunodeficiency disease (SCID)

Possibly an inherited disorder (autosomal recessive and X-linked recessive patterns of inheritance have been identified), SCID results in dysfunction of the production of antibody and complement and in all mediated immunity. Because of this immunodeficiency, children with SCID have an overwhelming susceptibility to infection and the graft-versus-host reaction.

Usually, susceptibility to infection occurs early in the affected infant's life. Infections tend to become chronic, resulting in the child's failure to thrive because of the frequent and persistent bouts of illness. If the child receives foreign tissue, such as a blood transfusion, the tissue damage initiates symptoms that may be mistaken for infection, further increasing the child's susceptibility.

Wiskott-Aldrich syndrome, an X-linked recessive disorder characterized by selective immunodeficiencies, eczema, and thrombocytopenia, has nursing guidelines similar to those of SCID. Carrier detection is available.

Assessment

Frequently encountered data for SCID include the following:

Subjective

• history of repeated infections and failure to ever recover completely

Objective

• signs and symptoms of infection, including fever, anorexia, malaise, irritability, listlessness, nausea, vomiting, diarrhea, lymphadenopathy, skin lesions, and change in body fluids
• symptoms of failure to thrive, such as altered growth and development.

Nursing diagnosis

Ineffective Family Coping related to guilt feelings associated with a genetic disease or disorder with life-threatening implications
Desired outcome: The caregivers demonstrate supportive, nurturing behaviors to supply the child's physical, psychosocial, and intellectual needs.

Interventions

1. Assess the caregiver-child relationship and contrast it to a desirable interaction.
2. Listen to the caregiver's expression of feelings.
3. Encourage the caregiver to seek the support of family, friends, and clergy.
4. Provide the opportunity for caregivers to interact with others in similar situations (such as parent support groups).
5. Supply caregiver guidelines (through literature and discus-

sions) that will provide the child with optimum security, self-esteem, and comfort.

6. Model appropriate relationships that fulfill the child's psychosocial needs (according to the child's developmental level). (Adults caring for terminally ill children may be inclined to allow manipulation and demanding behavior, although this type of behavior does not satisfy the child's needs.)

Medical diagnosis

The medical diagnosis for SCID is based on:
• history of recurrent, severe infections from early infancy
• familial history of the disorder
• laboratory findings, including lymphopenia, lack of lymphocyte response to antigens, and absence of plasma cells in bone marrow.

Medical treatment

Treatment includes:
• histocompatible bone marrow transplantation
• administration of immune globulin to provide passive immunity
• environmental control
• genetic counseling.

3 Trauma, Abuse, and Neglect

During your rotation on the pediatric unit, you'll likely encounter children with conditions resulting from trauma, abuse, or neglect. This section provides specific information on some of the major traumatic problems of childhood as well as on child abuse and neglect.

Although children of all age-groups encounter traumatic problems, young children (particularly infants and toddlers) are more at risk for diseases and disorders resulting from trauma. Below is a listing of some of the most commonly encountered trauma-related problems.

☐ Burns

One of the major causes of accidental death during childhood (leading causes include automobile accidents and drownings), burn injuries occur to children of all ages; however, about 70% of all pediatric burn injuries affect children under age 5.

Although accidents occur in even the most desirable of home environments, the incidence increases in environments in which children are less supervised or exposed to emotional disturbances within the family.

Because severe burns initiate a pathologic state in other body organs, nursing care presents a great challenge. The ultimate goals include preserving life, preventing infection, and promoting healing through emotional and physical rehabilitation.

If a burn victim has not completed the growth period (as with younger children), long-term care must include periodic releases of tissue contractures that limit mobility and increase disfigurement. The primary objectives of such care include the child's obtaining functional use of the burned areas and a cosmetic outcome that is as near to normal as is possible.

Assessment
First determine the depth of burn, as outlined below:
• First degree: Involves only the epidermis, which is reddened.
• Second degree (partial-thickness): Involves the epidermis and dermis, both the superficial and deep dermal layers; deep dermal layer may not be painful for 1 to 2 days after injury; blister formation appears on the reddened region.
• Third degree (full-thickness): Involves the entire dermis and penetrates into subcutaneous tissue; characterized by a brown leathery appearance.
• Fourth degree: Involves fascia, muscle, and perhaps bone.

Note: Evaluating the depth of the burn may be difficult immediately after injury. Frequently, varying degrees are involved. Next, determine the percentage of body surface burned. Age-related charts may be used to describe the percentage of total body surface area involved; body proportions vary at different ages (see *Distribution of burns in children by body surface area*).

Because of the extremely complex needs of the burn victim, the patient usually is admitted to a specialized unit or a burn hospital.

Nursing diagnosis

Fluid Volume Deficit and Electrolyte Imbalance related to loss of body fluid from denuded surfaces and blood loss from leakage of damaged capillaries

Desired outcome: The child receives adequate fluid and electrolyte replacement as evidenced by usual mental status, stable vital signs, balanced intake and output, and the absence of nausea, vomiting, muscle weakness, and other symptoms of imbalance. (See "Fluid and Electrolyte Imbalance" in the Appendices.)

Interventions

1. Monitor the child for signs and symptoms of hypovolemia, including decreased blood pressure, increased pulse and respiratory rates, and mental changes.
2. Insert an indwelling (Foley) catheter to monitor urine output (minimum amount 0.5 to 1 ml/kg/hour).
3. Monitor the child's body weight as related to a baseline weight.
4. Maintain I.V. fluid therapy, taking great care not to overload the child.
5. Assist with applying an occlusive or a biological dressing to reduce fluid loss through evaporation.
6. Maintain a constant environmental temperature; prevent drafts and chilling.
7. Encourage the child to verbalize fear and anxiety, which may be the cause of increased nausea and vomiting.
8. Respond to the child's needs as promptly as possible.

Nursing diagnosis

Impaired Skin Integrity related to injury, debridement and grafting procedures, delayed healing (caused by malnutrition, infection, or a high glucocorticoid level resulting from pain and stress), or decreased tissue perfusion (specify)

Desired outcome: The child experiences healing of the burn, graft, and donor sites as evidenced by granulation tissue in the wound, intact skin edges, and diminishing redness and discomfort.

Interventions

1. Monitor the child for signs and symptoms of impaired healing,

DISTRIBUTION OF BURNS IN CHILDREN BY BODY SURFACE AREA

To quickly estimate the extent of a child's burns, add up the percentages of body surface areas affected using the illustrations and corresponding charts below. The total percentage can be used to determine the child's initial fluid replacement needs.

Birth to age 9

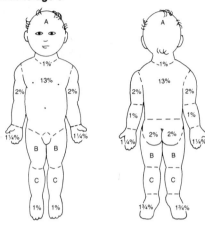

Percentage of body surface area (BSA) burned		
Birth to age 9		
Age	**BSA**	**Percent-age**
Birth to 12 months	A	9½%
	B	2¾%
	C	2½%
1 to 4 years	A	8½%
	B	3¼%
	C	2½%
5 to 9 years	A	6½%
	B	4%
	C	2¾%
Age 10 to adult		
Age	**BSA**	**Percent-age**
10 to 14 years	A	5½%
	B	4½%
	C	3%
15 to 17 years	A	4½%
	B	4½%
	C	3¼%
18 and older	A	3½%
	B	4¾%
	C	3½%

Age 10 to adult

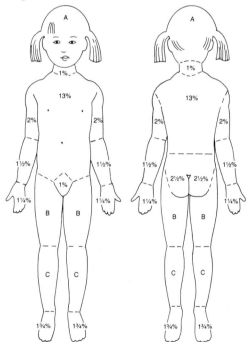

**Key: A = front or back of head
B = front or back of thigh
C = front or back of lower leg**

including redness, edema, purulent exudate, foul odor, increased amount of necrotic tissue, and separated graft edges. Also monitor for signs and symptoms of Curling's ulcer.

2. Implement measures to prevent wound infection, such as:
• using protective isolation precautions, including a gown, cap, mask, and sterile gloves, when handling the wound area
• preventing the child from coming in contact with persons with respiratory or skin infections
• providing wound care (covered or closed method) with scrupulous use of sterile technique and supplies. (Use bed cradles to keep bed linens from disturbing the healing process.)

3. Implement nutritional support. Initially, the child may be tube-fed or receive total parenteral nutrition. When oral intake is allowed, take the following measures to improve the child's nutritional status:
• Administer medication to reduce the child's pain.
• Provide oral care before meals.
• Serve at more frequent intervals small portions of food and fluid that are attractive to the child and of optimum nutritional value.
• Schedule wound care, range-of-motion exercises, or other painful procedures at least 1 hour before and after meals.
• Encourage rest or quiet diversionary activities before mealtime.
• Remain with the child during the meal to provide companionship and to divert his attention from feeding problems (even after the child can manage self-feeding).

4. Implement measures and treatments to provide adequate respiratory function, such as:
• deep breathing, coughing, and using an inspiratory exerciser every 2 hours
• turning and position changes (use semi-Fowler's if not contraindicated)
• assisting with postural drainage and chest physiotherapy, if ordered
• maintaining humidification devices
• administering medication to liquefy secretions.

Nursing diagnosis

Anxiety related to the effects of sudden injury on appearance and function, the unfamiliar environment of the hospital, and pain resulting from the injury and therapeutic procedures
Desired outcome: The child experiences reduced anxiety as evidenced by relaxed facial expressions and body language, verbalization of greater comfort, and verbalization of an understanding of the purpose for supplies and procedures involved in management.

Interventions

1. Orient the child to the hospital environment, routine, and equipment.

2. Maintain consistency in staff assignment.

3. Encourage discussion of fears and the reason for procedures.

4. Explain all assessment procedures, treatments, and diagnostic tests before initiating them, using diagrams and representative equipment to clarify and increase understanding. (Communication is the beginning of understanding. Include caregivers in all discussions and care when not contraindicated; the impact caused by disfigurement of the child may be overwhelming to caregivers.)

5. Administer pain medication before dressing changes, tub baths, and debridement. (The child will develop trust in the nurse who anticipates the pain involved in treatments.)

6. Encourage the child to assume self-care gradually, as much as possible. (Fear and anxiety diminish with redevelopment of self-confidence.)

Medical diagnosis

The medical diagnosis is based on an assessment of the percentage of body surface burned and on the depth and location of the burn. Systemic responses may lead to burn shock, anemia, acute renal failure, a greatly increased metabolic rate, increased adrenal activity, and a degree of metabolic acidosis.

Medical treatment

In planning the medical treatment of the burned patient, the following factors are considered:

• the amount of tissue destroyed

• the child's age (children under age 2 have a higher mortality than older children)

• the cause of the injury (thermal, chemical, or electrical)

• the extent of damage to the respiratory system (Maintaining an open airway is essential to survival.)

• the child's health status before the injury

• other injury.

See *Burn care methods: Advantages and disadvantages,* page 198, for details on specific treatments.

Emergency care

Emergency treatment includes:

• stopping the burning process

• covering the burn with a clean cloth to minimize contamination and pain (from air contact)

• providing I.V. fluid therapy and oxygen to prevent burn shock

• providing psychological support by reassuring the child (and caregivers) so that additional coping with the psychological stress may not cause an overload on the stress mechanism of the body, which is challenged by the physical injury.

BURN CARE METHODS: ADVANTAGES AND DISADVANTAGES

Exposure therapy

After the wound is cleansed, it is exposed to air and allowed to dry. This promotes formation of a natural protective barrier from the hardened coagulum of exudate (partial-thickness burns) or from dry eschar (full-thickness burns).

Advantages
• Does not require bulky dressings
• Permits frequent inspection
• Produces less odor
• Ensures less fluid loss during the initial phases
• Acts as a poor culture medium for bacteria because of crust formation

Disadvantages
• Allows for greater risk of cross-contamination
• Requires strict isolation technique
• Requires maintaining optimum environmental temperature
• Frequently requires placing restraints on the child's extremities (to prevent picking at crusted areas)
• Presents an unsightly appearance

Occlusive dressings

The wound's inner layer is covered with an even layer of absorptive, resilient, fluffed gauze that is held in place with nonconstricting stretch gauze bandages. The wound surface is covered with nonadherent, water-permeable fin-mesh gauze.

Advantages
• Provides protection from injury and cross-contamination
• Permits better mobilization
• Aids in positioning and resting injured area
• Produces less pain initially

Disadvantages
• Requires skilled nursing care
• Associated with a higher incidence of hyperpyrexia
• Maintains a warm, moist environment conducive to bacterial growth
• Frequently requires pain medication (dressing changes may be uncomfortable)

Primary excision

This method involves the immediate surgical excision of devitalizing tissue followed by grafting.

Advantages
• Provides a permanent replacement for damaged tissue
• Reduces exposure to wound infection

Disadvantages
• Makes it difficult to distinguish between full-thickness and partial-thickness injuries
• Associated with significant blood loss

Minor burns

Treatment for minor burns includes:
• cleansing and debriding the wound (using nonirritating soap and a sterile saline rinse and covering the wound with a bulky gauze dressing to protect the child from trauma)
• possibly using antiseptic or antimicrobial cream
• splinting burns on hands and feet to prevent deformity
• administering tetanus antitoxin, if indicated by the patient's history
• administering pain medication, such as acetaminophen
• changing dressing to debride, prevent infection, and promote healing.

Major burns

Treatment for major burns includes:
• establishing and maintaining the child's airway, using:
  —oxygen, a Croupette, or an Oxyhood to manage humidity
  —an endotracheal tube if symptoms of air hunger are observed
  —a tracheostomy (if needed)

—a nasogastric tube to prevent tachypnea resulting from acute gastric dilation and vomiting (Paralytic ileus is not uncommon in children.)

• instituting fluid replacement therapy to:
—compensate for body fluid lost from trauma
—restore plasma volume
—obtain adequate perfusion and correct acidosis
—provide nutrients in response to high metabolic requirements (I.V. hyperalimentation or nasogastric tube feeding)

• administering medication (Analgesics and sedatives are essential; use of prophylactic antibiotics or heparin depends on the specific circumstances.)

• providing care of the burn wound by use of exposure therapy, occlusive dressings, or primary excision. (Full-thickness wound care focuses on preventing infection, the removal of dead tissue, protecting the child from mechanical trauma, and closure of the wound.)

☐ Craniocerebral trauma

Craniocerebral trauma usually results from falls or accidental bumping of the head. Head injury may be classified as mild, moderate, or severe (see *Classifying closed head injuries,* page 201). The specific treatment and prognosis depend on the area involved and the severity of trauma.

The head is extremely vulnerable to injury because of its exposed nature; the immature skull can sustain greater impact without fracture. Most children "bump" their heads sometime during the growing-up years; thousands are admitted to the hospital each year for evaluation and treatment. Lacerations of the scalp usually prompt caregivers to seek medical attention.

Assessment

Frequently encountered data for craniocerebral trauma include the following:

Subjective

Based on a detailed history of the events surrounding the injury, findings may include headache (may be identified by behavioral changes, such as irritability and refusal to alter position).

Objective

• alterations in consciousness (confusion, somnolence, listlessness, or change in behavior)
• vomiting (noting the type [such as projectile], frequency, and amount)
• rise in systolic blood pressure with widening pulse pressure
• full, bounding, slow pulse
• pupillary response changes (poorly reactive to light and accommodation, lack of consensual response)

• constant headache aggravated by movement
• bleeding or watery discharge from the nose or ears (discharge that tests positive for glucose [using a Dextrostix], possibly indicating cerebrospinal fluid leakage)
• motor changes (muscular weakness to paralysis)
• sensory changes (such as numbness)
• reflex changes
• seizure activity.

Nursing diagnosis

Ineffective Family Coping related to fear, anxiety, temporary changes in the child's motor and sensory function, and mental confusion

Desired outcome: The child and caregivers cope with the situation as evidenced by verbalization of feelings and relaxed body language.

Interventions

1. Orient the child and caregivers to the hospital environment, equipment, and routines.
2. Maintain consistency in the nursing staff to provide a feeling of stability and comfort.
3. Encourage verbalization of fears and provide feedback.
4. Explain all diagnostic tests before they are performed.
5. Reinforce the doctor's explanations and attempt to clarify any misunderstanding.
6. Reassure the child that temporary changes in his function do not necessarily indicate a long-term problem.
7. Include the child and caregivers in the care plan and allow choices when possible.

Nursing diagnosis

Altered Tissue Perfusion, Cerebral: Decreased Physiologic or Behavioral Responsiveness related to the effects of the development of increased intracranial pressure (ICP)

Desired outcome: The child does not develop increased ICP as evidenced by his usual or improved level of consciousness, stable vital signs, and neurologic assessment. Or, if the nurse identifies signs and symptoms of increased ICP, early medical-surgical intervention prevents further damage.

Interventions

1. Take appropriate measures to maximize the child's ability to cope, thereby lessening his stress reaction.
2. Monitor the child for signs and symptoms of increased ICP (may be necessary to arouse the child every 15 minutes during the acute phase).
3. Restrict fluids to include clear liquids only; administer fluids at an even rate, according to doctor's orders.
4. Measure the child's intake and output.

CLASSIFYING CLOSED HEAD INJURIES

Type of injury	Defining characteristics
Minor (cerebral concussion)	• Causes transient and reversible damage to nerve cells and fibers • Results in a momentary to brief lapse of consciousness followed by a rapid return to a normal level of alertness and amnesia of the incident • Produces no abnormal neurologic symptoms
Moderate (cerebral contusion)	• Causes damage to larger areas (with small petechial hemorrhages and edema at the injury site and the area directly opposite the injury) • Results in a longer period of unconsciousness • May cause focal disturbances and lack of nerve function in the bruised area (temporal lobe)
Severe (brain stem contusion)	• Causes damage to the upper brain stem, causing compression of the reticular activating system (which controls the level of consciousness) and the corticospinal tracts, resulting in motor abnormalities of the face and extremities • Results in immediate onset of coma (improvement is extremely gradual) • May cause neurologic abnormalities (initially on the same side as the injury), such as dilated pupils
Severe (cerebral lacerations)	• Causes tears and severe bleeding in and around the tears • Associated with penetrating injuries and depressed skull fracture • May cause neurologic abnormalities • Results in permanent scarring of the injured area with some degree of disability

5. Elevate the head of the bed 20 to 30 degrees unless contraindicated.

6. Avoid neck flexion positioning.

7. Provide a quiet environment to reduce restlessness and irritability.

8. Instruct the child about the need for bed rest and for additional safety measures, such as side rails.

9. Observe the child for unusual behavior.

10. Encourage the caregivers to remain at the bedside to provide valuable information on changes from the child's norm.

11. If the patient is an infant, measure the head circumference and check the size and tension of fontanelles.

Medical diagnosis

The medical diagnosis is based on:

• the clinical examination
• skull X-rays
• EEG readings
• brain scan, echoencephalography, and cerebral angiography
• computed tomography scan
• lumbar puncture (rarely done when increased ICP is suspected)

• subdural tap through the fontanelle or coronal suture (to diagnose subdural or epidermal hemorrhage).

Medical treatment
Treatment includes:
• continued observation and reevaluation of the child's status if the early condition reveals no serious injury
• administering I.V. fluids at a minimal rate to keep the vein open (Avoid overhydration and aggravating cerebral edema by using one half the normal volume.)
• administering clear liquids by mouth or giving nothing by mouth
• administering anticonvulsants for seizures or when a contusion or laceration is suspected
• administering hypertonic solutions and osmotic diuretics (mannitol) for cerebral edema
• providing tepid sponge baths or a hypothermia blanket for hyperthermia
• surgical reduction for depressed fractures
• administering sedatives for restlessness cautiously to avoid masking signs and symptoms of increased ICP.

☐ Failure to thrive

A condition in which a child's weight or height (or both) consistently falls below the third percentile, failure to thrive (FTT) is characterized by inadequate caloric intake, retention, or use (or possibly a combination of all three). Without intervention, the disorder may become chronic and life-threatening. About 80% of all reported cases involve children under age 18 months.

Existing in all social classes, FTT may be classified according to one of three etiologic categories: organic, nonorganic, or mixed. Organic FTT results from a disease or disorder, such as chronic heart failure, renal insufficiency, cystic fibrosis, malabsorption syndrome, or an endocrine disorder. Nonorganic FTT, not associated with any diagnosed disease or disorder, usually involves a psychosocial problem between the child and primary caregiver. Mixed FTT results from a combination of organic and nonorganic causes.

Early in the assessment process, nonorganic FTT should be considered to prevent subjecting the child to the trauma of diagnostic procedures. Contributing factors of nonorganic FTT may include emotional nonfulfillment of the expectations of the infant or caregivers and physical or psychosocial conditions. Although maternal deprivation syndrome has been used to describe the problem, the term caregiver-child attachment deprivation syndrome may be more appropriate.

Caregivers at increased risk for attachment problems commonly have the following associated characteristics:

• isolation and social crises
• inadequate support systems
• lack of education
• physical or mental health problems (or both), possibly including drug dependence, depression, or retardation
• immaturity (especially with adolescent parents)
• a lack of commitment to parenting.

Assessment
Frequently encountered data for FTT include the following:

Subjective
• history of difficult feeding (including poor appetite, poor sucking reflex, crying during feeding, and vomiting)
• irregular pattern in daily living (usually resulting from disharmony between the child's and caregivers' temperaments)

Objective
• signs and symptoms of malnutrition (based on weight below the third percentile for the child's age or less than 80% of ideal weight for age and on an estimate of total body fat)
• body language (stiff, unpliable, and rigid or "floppy" infant; gaze avoidance; lack of molding between caregiver's and child's body)
• observation of feeding patterns, including:
    —the infant's behavior indicating hunger
    —the position assumed by the infant when held
    —sucking behavior (response to nipple or spoon)
    —eye-to-eye contact
    —the infant's response to stimuli, such as stroking or cuddling
    —the amount of food ingested
    —the time taken for feeding
• observation of the caregiver's reaction to the infant's needs.

Nursing diagnosis
Altered Nutrition: Less Than Body Requirements related to effect of organic disorders or nonorganic factors, such as neglect
Desired outcome: The child has a weight gain of (specify)____ lb within (specify) _____.

Interventions
1. Assess the child for difficulties during feeding time, such as poor sucking, crying, and aversion behavior.
2. Limit feeding to as few staff as possible; agree on a similar approach to mealtimes and be consistent.
3. Make feeding a priority; schedule other activities and procedures so that the atmosphere remains calm, relaxed, and pain-free.
4. Keep an accurate record of the child's intake (calorie count).
5. Weigh the child daily at the same time and with the same clothing.

6. Hold the infant or young child during feeding.

7. Precede feeding with close physical and eye contract to stimulate interest in the relationship.

8. Talk to the child during feeding.

9. Follow the child's natural rhythm in eating.

10. Observe the child's food preferences; serve palatable, appealing foods to the child who is old enough for solids.

11. Praise the child for accomplishments at the end of the meal.

12. Gradually integrate the caregiver into the feeding process.

Nursing diagnosis

Altered Growth and Development related to inadequate provision of the infant's or child's basic needs by the caregiver

Desired outcome: The child has improved growth and development as evidenced by age-appropriate appetite, less stiffness or flaccidity in physical contact, rhythmicity in sleeping, interest in surroundings, and more responsive facial expressions.

Interventions

1. Ensure continuity of care through consistent assignment of nursing staff.

2. Assess the child's developmental status.

3. Observe the child's patterns of seeking attention, comfort, and provision of basic needs.

4. Establish a routine of care modified by cues taken from the child.

5. Handle the child with gentle confidence.

6. Use eye-to-eye contact with child.

7. Talk to the child during caregiving, confirming his presence.

8. Use physical contact, such as hugging, rocking, cuddling, and stroking, as much as possible; continue with this approach even though the child may resist it initially.

9. Schedule time for the child to be with a child-life specialist for playroom activities.

10. Provide at the bedside toys that are appropriate for the child's developmental level.

Nursing diagnosis

Anxiety (Parental) related to the child's lack of normal growth and development

Desired outcome: The caregivers participate in providing appropriate care.

Interventions

1. Establish lines of communication with the caregivers.

2. Encourage caregivers to express feelings and beliefs about their lives and parenting.

3. Discuss the caregiver-child relationship and emphasize the caregivers' previous success in relating themselves to the child.

4. Demonstrate how to perceive the child's cues for attention by

providing examples during actual care of the child—whether care is tendered by the nurse or by the caregiver with the nurse at the bedside.
5. Provide literature on parenting skills, including anticipatory guidance.
6. Affirm the assistance given by official agencies and parent support groups.
7. Remain at the bedside while the caregiver feeds the child, provides hygiene needs, and plays with the child to encourage and praise successful interaction.

Medical diagnosis

The medical diagnosis for FTT is based on:
• the patient history
• assessment of the child's developmental status, including results of the Denver Developmental Screening Test
• acknowledgment of risk factors
• diagnostic tests and procedures, as indicated, to identify organic diseases or disorders
• assessment of the child's feeding.

Medical treatment

Treatment includes:
• appropriate treatment of an organic problem to minimize its effect on development
• nurturing of the entire family to establish emotional, physical, and developmental health
• opportunity for caregivers to improve their own self-esteem and improve parenting skills (group and individual counseling classes)
• use of substitute caregivers (such as the nursing staff) to change feeding habit patterns
• continued ongoing assessment
• increasing the child's calorie intake within a determined volume of feeding (for example, giving 24, 27, or 30 calories/oz) and adding fat sources (such as corn oil) and carbohydrates (such as Polycose Glucose Polymer) to the diet.

☐ Foreign body ingestion, aspiration, or insertion

Foreign bodies or materials may be ingested, aspirated, or become lodged in the passageways of infants and young children. Curious about objects, children under age 3 typically explore their environment by putting foreign materials in their mouths or pushing them into their nostrils or ear canals.

Children, especially those weakened by illness, are prone to aspiration of regurgitated food, fluid, or secretions. Swallowed items (such as coins, buttons, small rocks, safety pins, and toy parts) usually pass through the GI tract without causing damage.

Occasionally, however, an item becomes lodged in one place and sometimes perforates the wall of the gut. For this reason, all persons caring for children must be prepared to recognize when aspiration has occurred and to intervene promptly.

Pathologic changes caused by aspiration may result from occlusion of the bronchi or bronchioles by the foreign body or from resultant inflammation and edema of the mucosa. Atelectasis, emphysema, inflammation, or abscess may develop. Specifically, aspirated petroleum distillates cause severe pneumonia; aspirated gastric contents cause toxic effects to the airways and alveoli; and aspirated dry vegetable matter, which may expand when moist, may be difficult to remove.

Assessment
Frequently encountered data for foreign body ingestion, aspiration, or insertion include the following:

Subjective
• history of the missing item
• pain or discomfort
• description of the gagging or choking episode
• history of persistent respiratory infection

Objective
Signs of the lodging of the item in the following body parts:
Larynx
• hoarseness, croupy cough, and inability to speak
• hemoptysis
• dyspnea
• cyanosis
Trachea
• cough
• hoarseness
• dyspnea with asthmatic wheeze
• cyanosis
Bronchi
(depends on degree of blockage of the passageway)
• limited expansion of the lungs
• diminished breath sounds (atelectasis)
• signs and symptoms of pneumonia with fever and purulent sputum
Nasal cavity
• bloody or purulent, foul-smelling nasal discharge
External auditory canal
• earache
• drainage from ear canal
GI tract
• abdominal pain
• fever

• abdominal distention to rigidity (boardlike abdomen) and other symptoms of intestinal perforation.

Nursing diagnosis

(*Note:* The nursing care of pneumonia, bronchitis, or intestinal symptoms after the aspiration or ingestion of a foreign body is similar to care given for conditions initiated by other etiologies, such as microorganisms or an incarcerated hernia.)
Ineffective Airway Clearance related to obstruction
Desired outcome: The child has breath sounds and no signs of choking.

Interventions

1. Recognize the following symptoms of choking:
• inability to speak or cry
• cyanosis
• collapse.
2. Initiate an obstructed airway maneuver (see Section 5).
3. Prevent aspiration from regurgitation by positioning the infant or weak or comatose child on his side or abdomen after feeding.
4. Elevate the child to a semi-Fowler's position on his right side if not contraindicated.
5. Teach the caregivers to monitor the child's environment.
6. Eliminate potential hazards, such as balloons, from the child's environment; check toys for small, potentially removable parts.
7. Do not allow the small child to eat popcorn, nuts, potato chips, or unpeeled hot dogs.
8. If vomiting occurs, hold the infant upside down; keep the older child's head lower than his chest or position his head between his legs.

Medical diagnosis

The medical diagnosis is based on:
• identification of the causative agent by observing the aspirated contents and oral secretions for a food item (such as a peanut, seed, or piece of popcorn) or foreign object (such as a coin or toy part) or liquid substance (such as petroleum distillate)
• the patient history and physical findings
• X-ray
• fluoroscopy
• bronchoscopy
• otoscopic examination.

Medical treatment

Treatment includes:
• first-aid for a choking child (see Section 5)
• removal of the foreign material from the child's airway as soon as possible by laryngoscopy or bronchoscopy
• after removal of the foreign material, placing the child in a Croupette to facilitate movement of air in small, edematous pas-

sageways and treating or preventing pneumonia with antibiotics
• if the material was ingested, following the passage of the item through the GI tract by X-ray or fluoroscopy
• examining the stool to retrieve the object
• if the foreign material is lodged in the child's ear or nose, removing the object and administering antibiotic therapy if infection has developed.

☐ Poisoning

Children will swallow almost anything, even poisonous substances. Most poisonings occur at about age 2, when the toddler gains more independence in mobility, explores his environment, and has poor discriminatory taste. Although many children die from accidental poisoning, many more survive with residual damage, such as esophageal stricture or damage to the kidneys or liver.

Usually, by the time the child is admitted to the pediatric unit, the poison has been identified and exposure to the substance alleviated. Emergency treatment includes induction of vomiting (except in cases involving ingestion of petroleum distillates or caustic substances, such as lye, and loss of the gag reflex) or gastric lavage.

Specific toxins require specific treatment. Depending on the child's status, prompt intervention may focus on providing respiratory or circulatory (shock) assistance or control of seizures. Interventions related to shock include elevating the child's legs, applying warmth externally, promoting physical and mental rest (through calm reassurance from the staff), and maintaining quiet surroundings. In some cases, mouth-to-mouth resuscitation or insertion of an endotracheal tube for mechanical ventilation may be necessary.

Usually, the caregivers experience an emotional crisis from guilt, fear, and loss of self-confidence in parenting. Be careful not to appear judgmental or to initiate teaching to prevent recurrence until the child is well on the road to recovery. A home evaluation should follow any admission for poisoning to assist caregivers with awareness and prevention.

Assessment

Frequently encountered data for poisoning include the following:

Acetaminophen
• within 2 to 24 hours after ingestion:
— nausea and vomiting
— anorexia
— sweating and pallor
• after 24 to 36 hours (and lasting 6 to 8 days):

—evidence of liver damage, including jaundice and neuromuscular and mental changes related to hepatic coma

Acids and alkalis
• corrosion of mucous membranes of the mouth, throat, and esophagus
• abdominal pain
• intense thirst with difficulty in swallowing
• diarrhea
• shallow, dyspneic respirations

Hydrocarbons
• cough
• dyspnea and cyanosis
• symptoms of pneumonitis

Lead (plumbism)
• pica (including eating dirt, ashes, paint chips, paper, crayons, and cigarette butts)
• anemia-related fatigue
• anorexia
• pallor
• irritability
• glycosuria, proteinuria, and ketonuria
• central nervous system–related hyperactivity
• delayed or regressed speech
• loss of motor abilities
• learning problems
• convulsions
• coma
• death

Salicylates
• mild toxicity
• tinnitus
• dizziness
• sweating
• nausea and vomiting
• diarrhea
• delirium
• severe toxicity
• hyperventilation
• high fever
• acidosis and electrolyte imbalance
• tremors
• bleeding
• convulsions
• cerebral hemorrhage
• coma.

Nursing diagnosis (for ingestion of salicylates or acetaminophen in toxic amounts)

Potential for Injury related to the effects of drug toxicity
Desired outcome: The child has no signs or symptoms of drug toxicity after treatment.

Interventions

1. Recognize the signs and symptoms of toxicity (as indicated under "Assessment").
2. Induce vomiting by administering ipecac syrup.
3. Assist with gastric lavage, as ordered.
4. Administer I.V. fluids and electrolytes, as ordered.
5. Monitor the child's intake and output; check urine specific gravity.
6. Monitor the child's vital signs frequently (every 15 minutes initially).
7. Reduce fever with tepid sponge baths or a cooling blanket.
8. Initiate seizure precautions; administer anticonvulsants as necessary.
9. Observe for bleeding.
10. Explain all procedures to the child and caregivers before beginning the intervention.
11. Avoid reinforcing child or parental guilt by asking them to repeat the history.
12. After the acute phase, provide prevention information.

Nursing diagnosis (for lead poisoning [plumbism])

Potential for Injury related to the effects of excess lead deposited in the tissues (hematologic, renal, or central nervous system)
Desired outcome: The child recovers from the toxic condition as evidenced by urine and blood analysis and clinical observations.

Interventions

1. Assist with collection of specimens for blood lead levels and erythrocyte protoporphyrin and urinary coproporphyrin levels.
2. Explain the reason for the tests to the child and caregivers.
3. Prepare the child for administration of multiple, painful injections using play therapy.
4. Plan a systematic rotation of injection sites; explain this to the caregivers.
5. Use large muscle groups, such as the vastus lateralis, ventrogluteal, and gluteal sites for injections. (Check that the gluteus is sufficiently developed.)
6. Feel the muscle before injecting medication to check for fibrous changes (such as a hard, painful lump) from previous injections.
7. If ordered, use procaine in the injection to lessen pain. (Draw the chelating agent [viscous solution] into the syringe first; follow this with the anesthetic so that the anesthetic will be injected

first. Use an air bubble in the syringe to flush the needle of medication and decrease the risk of tracking painful medication through tissue as the needle is withdrawn.)

8. Schedule activities to allow meals and rest time between injections.

9. Apply warm soaks or heating pads to injection sites.

10. Avoid having the child use painful muscles. (For example, use a wheelchair or provide quiet play activities suitable to the child's developmental level.)

11. Encourage fluid intake; maintain an I.V. line, if ordered.

12. Measure the child's intake and output.

13. Implement seizure precautions; keep suction and airway equipment readily accessible.

14. Monitor for seizures and alert caregivers to the possibility of their occurrence.

15. Provide emotional support to the child and caregivers during difficult courses of treatment.

Nursing diagnosis (for lead poisoning [plumbism])
Potential for Injury: Poisoning related to increased risk of return to previous behaviors and environment
Desired outcome: The child's lead levels remain at low risk as evidenced by blood lead concentrations and erythrocyte-protoporphyrin levels.

Interventions
1. Discuss the danger of lead ingestion with the caregivers.

2. Relate the need for prevention to the painful treatment needed to eliminate lead from body tissue.

3. Explore ways of decreasing the child's pica behavior by providing stimulating activities.

4. Assist with referral to social service agencies to evaluate the home environment and the family's socioeconomic needs.

5. Suggest the use of support systems (family, friends, and community groups) in times of stress or crisis.

6. Provide written materials affirming the need for public education.

Medical diagnosis
The medical diagnosis for poisoning is based on the patient history and the following:
Acetaminophen
• serum acetaminophen levels
• liver and renal function tests
Acids and alkalis
• analysis of the causative agent (such as lye or bleach)
Hydrocarbons
• identification of additional toxic agents (such as pesticides)
• chest X-ray
• monitoring of signs and symptoms of chemical pneumonitis

Lead
- physical examination
- blood lead concentrations
- erythrocyte protoporphyrin levels
- 24-hour urine specimen for lead and evidence of renal damage
- X-rays for presence of lead chips in the GI tract

Salicylates
- serum salicylate levels (peak in 2 to 4 hours after ingestion).
- determination of degree of toxicity through use of a nomogram (salicylate level related to time of ingestion).

Medical treatment
Treatment includes the following:

Acetaminophen
- removal of drug by emesis or gastric lavage
- administration of an antidote (acetylcysteine); because of the antidote's offensive smell, a nasogastric tube may be used

Acids and alkalis
- avoidance of a lavage tube or an emetic
- dilution of the causative agent with water (*Note:* Attempts to neutralize acids or alkalis may cause greater damage or obscure membranes for assessment.)
- maintenance of a patent airway
- administration of a pain medication
- long-term care (possibly including methods to prevent esophageal stricture, such as dilation [after the acute period] or surgery for stenosis [later])

Hydrocarbons
- prevention of aspiration
- avoidance of inducing vomiting
- use of gastric lavage (especially if another toxin is involved)
- administration of steroids for inflammation
- administration of antibiotics for secondary bacterial infection

Lead
- depending on the severity of poisoning, chelation therapy (administration of edetate disodium to increase urinary excretion of lead and dimercaprol to remove lead from the nervous system; may involve six injections per day for 5 days)
- control of seizures (see "Seizures" under the "Neuromuscular and musculoskeletal systems" heading in Section 2)
- blood replacement (for severe anemia) and occasionally exchange transfusions
- administration of enemas to remove lead from the GI tract

Salicylates
- forced emesis or gastric lavage
- administration of activated charcoal
- administration of electrolytes I.V. for acid-base imbalance
- administration of I.V. fluids to facilitate excretion
- administration of calories and fluids to compensate for in-

creased metabolic rate
- vitamin K to decrease bleeding potential
- use of dialysis (if condition is life-threatening).

☐ Spinal cord injury

Although cord injury is not a common cause of neurologic deficits in children, numerous types of accidents may result in compression, contusion, laceration, or severing of the tissue. Motor vehicle accidents (including automobiles and bicycles), sports-related injuries (from participation in football, diving, or gymnastics), and even gunshot wounds may initiate trauma to the cord. Most frequently, spinal cord injuries involve levels T12, L1, and C5 and C6 (or C1 and C2).

Cord injury without vertebral trauma is not uncommon in children because of the cartilaginous rings of the immature skeletal column. When trauma occurs at a high level, quadriplegia and physiologic deficits in most vital systems result from disruption of the central, peripheral, and autonomic nervous systems. Although advances in the immediate treatment of cord injury have improved the prognosis, the extent and severity of permanent deficits may not be known for several weeks.

The pathologic response to spinal cord injury may be described in stages. The first stage (spinal shock syndrome) is characterized by flaccid paralysis, loss of sensation and motor function, and impaired autonomic function as evidenced by loss of bladder and bowel control, hypotension, and alteration in body temperature in response to the environment.

In the second stage, spinal reflexes may cause extremity movements and spasticity from frequent contraction; in partial lesions, neurologic recovery may account for this activity. Autonomic dysreflexia occurs when sensory stimuli initiate responses without an inhibiting control. An extreme rise in blood pressure, possibly triggered by bladder and bowel distention, may lead to cerebrovascular accident, as manifested by flushing, headache, sweating, nasal stuffiness, goose bumps, and bradycardia. (Bladder and bowel distention must be prevented or treated.)

In the final stage, rehabilitation is based on maximizing the function regained through recovery. Infants and children with cord injury are much more vulnerable to spinal deformity than are those victims who have completed the growth phase. Immobilization or positioning devices may be used to limit this problem.

Assessment

Frequently encountered data for spinal cord injury include the following:

Subjective

- history of injury
- loss of sensation below the lesion

Objective
- absence of reflexes at or below the lesion
- loss of motor function with progressive atrophy
- initial muscle flaccidity (spasticity may develop later)
- alterations in body temperature
- hypotension
- respiratory distress (with high-level lesions)
- loss of bladder and bowel control
- atonic bladder with retention (hypertonic bladder may develop later).

Nursing diagnosis
(*Note:* Interventions frequently associated with spinal cord injury are complex and must be related to the stage of recovery, the potential for return of function or deficits [or both], and the child's developmental level. The outlook for the child is more positive if emotional adjustment is satisfactory and life-threatening consequences of urinary system abnormalities are avoided.)
Disturbance in Self-concept: Self-esteem and Personal Identity related to dependence on others to meet self-care needs
Desired outcome: The child will begin to assume control in achieving his potential for independence.

Interventions
1. Allow time for the child to adjust to his assets and deficits (the stages of the grieving process).
2. Encourage the child to verbalize feelings during this process.
3. Develop a rehabilitation program that includes management of mobility, exercise, skin care, nutrition, bowel and bladder control, education, and diversionary activity appropriate to the child's developmental level.
4. Include the child in the plan of care and in establishing the schedule of daily routine.
5. Demonstrate acceptance of alterations in body image by use of touch and humor.
6. Set realistic goals.
7. Expect the child to be "normal"; do not reinforce dependence by assuming that loss of control is unavoidable.
8. Use adaptive equipment, and brainstorm ways in which child can perform.
9. Provide privacy while the child is learning new tasks to avoid embarrassment.
10. Praise accomplishments.
11. Mainstream the child into the educational system.
12. Acknowledge threats to the child's self-concept according to his age and developmental stage (such as choice of a vocation and sexual development and awareness).

Nursing diagnosis
Urine Retention related to bladder or sphincter dysfunction (or both)

Desired outcome: The child experiences no urine retention or incomplete bladder emptying that may result in urinary tract infections, reflux, kidney damage, and sepsis.

Interventions

1. Monitor the child for signs and symptoms of urine retention, including suprapubic distention and imbalances in intake and output.
2. Insert and maintain a urinary catheter during spinal shock (paying particular attention to hygiene and tubing patency).
3. Use the following measures to promote complete bladder emptying after spinal shock:
• Stimulate the reflex sacral arc.
• Place the child in an upright position to void (if not contraindicated).
4. Continue to monitor for urine retention.
5. Perform intermittent catheterizations, as ordered.
6. Teach the child to perform self-catheterization.
7. Implement measures to promote urinary continence, when indicated.
8. Maintain consistent and adequate fluid intake to avoid overdistention of the bladder; however, limit evening intake (a bedtime incontinence risk).
9. Teach the use of trigger zones for reflex sacral arc.
10. Assess the quality of the child's urine.
11. Encourage mobility and upright posture to stimulate urine flow.
12. Administer urinary antiseptics, such as co-trimoxazole, and parasympathetic-blocking agents (to decrease hypertonicity and hyperreflexia).
13. Avoid the use of indwelling (Foley) catheters.

Medical diagnosis

The medical diagnosis for spinal cord injury is based on:
• the history of the accident
• a complete neurologic examination, including:
—reflex arcs
—sensory tracts related to stimulation of dermatone areas (body surface area that corresponds to spinal cord segment)
—voluntary motor function (with and without resistance and against gravity)
—degree of loss of autonomic innervations (vascular tone, body temperature regulation, and bowel and bladder regulation)
• X-ray to localize the lesion.

Medical treatment

Treatment includes:
• avoiding any twisting or bending of the spine

• initial use of emergency protocol to limit cord damage from edema
• cervical traction to prevent further neuronal damage (with high vertebral fractures)
• respiratory support (such as an endotracheal tube, a tracheostomy, or a ventilator)
• surgical intervention (occasionally)
• ideal rehabilitative treatment (using a team approach, such as a spinal injury center) to prevent complications and maximize functional abilities
• physical and occupational therapy.

☐ Child abuse and neglect

In recent years, the number of reported cases of child abuse has risen sharply. The majority of caregivers who maltreat their children by inflicting physical trauma, sexual molestation, or neglecting basic needs do not know—or cannot admit—that they are harming the child. Frequently, the abusive adult has been abused as a child. Some of these caregivers are aware of their actions but are afraid (or don't know how) to get help.

Because the abusive adult rarely seeks help for his own behavior, health care personnel must routinely observe and assess infants and children for signs and symptoms of parental or caretaker incompetence. Potential triggers for maltreatment include the caretaker, the child, and environmental factors.

The abusive caretaker may seek help for the child when trauma or neglect becomes a major threat. However, the caretaker may be so preoccupied with self-interests that, in the acute phase of the child's illness or injury, you may observe signs of distrust and hostility. In such a situation, your greatest nursing challenge may be to refrain from adopting a condemning attitude toward the abuser so you can achieve the best outcome for the child.

In the pediatric clinical setting, you'll need to remain open to behavioral clues and alert to evidence of potential or previous maltreatment so that appropriate interventions to prevent future harm may be initiated. In all states, ignoring the role of child advocate and not reporting suspected abuse or neglect to a child protection (or other) agency is considered a misdemeanor.

Assessment

The need for protective investigation into the child-caregiver relationship may be indicated by a combination of the many signs and symptoms of possible physical, emotional, or sexual abuse (including neglect).

Physical indications of possible abuse include bruises, welts, burns, fractures, dislocations, lacerations, and abrasions. These injuries may occur accidentally; however, their location, pattern, and frequency of occurrence may serve as clues to possible abuse.

Emotional indicators of possible abuse include withdrawal, fear of adult physical contact, antisocial behaviors, display of self-stimulating behaviors, slow social development, or unusual sophistication for the child's age.

Sexual abuse must be considered when the genital area is traumatized or infected. Indications of possible physical or emotional neglect include signs of failure to thrive, poor hygiene, and lack of health care or supervision.

Nursing diagnosis
Altered Parenting related to abuse as a child, poor self-image, lack of knowledge about normal developmental expectations, unsatisfied personal needs, or the inability to cope with life (perceived as a crisis)(specify)

Desired outcome: No further signs of physical punishment are evident, and parents show a willingness to participate in a therapy program. Also, the child's behavior remains within the norms for his developmental level.

Interventions
Prevention

1. During the prenatal care period, identify families at risk for abuse; observe the parents' attitude toward the pregnancy, availability of support systems, and future expectations of the caregiver-child relationship.
2. During well-infant or child checkups, identify families at risk by observing behaviors that reveal a lack of understanding of the child's needs, disappointment in the child's progress, and verbalization of a lack of support from family or friends.
3. Be a receptive listener.
4. Provide information on norms of growth and development (verbally and with literature).
5. Encourage the search for, and use of, support systems.
6. Encourage participation in parenting classes.
7. Demonstrate desirable interactions with the child and ways of handling developmental goals or problems.
8. Affirm the caregivers' use of effective behaviors with the child.

Protection

1. Orient caregivers to the hospital pediatric unit, and emphasize their importance to the child's care.
2. Identify and document any signs and symptoms of abuse or neglect, including the child's physical condition and behavior around the caregivers and others.
3. Report indicators of abuse or neglect through appropriate channels.
4. When discussing with the caregivers about the child's eventual

return home, recognize that their abusive behavior is unacceptable but stress that they have the potential for correcting the situation.

5. Encourage the caregivers to visit the child and to participate in his care as much as possible.

6. Affirm the outcome of individual therapy, family counseling, and close supervision by professionals, which should lead to a happier family unit.

7. Teach acceptable behavior through demonstration and role modeling.

Nursing diagnosis

Anxiety related to lack of an appropriate parental relationship and fear of maltreatment

Desired outcome: The child gains confidence in having basic needs met as evidenced by improved physical status (better appetite, sleep patterns, and progress toward developmental milestones) and behavioral patterns (reduction in self-stimulating behaviors, withdrawal, fearfulness, and disruptive behaviors).

Interventions

1. Provide consistency in assignment of the nursing staff.
2. Maintain protective measures for the hospitalized child.
3. Establish a routine of care for meals, play, and sleep.
4. Explain all procedures and treatments to the child so that invasive or painful events will not be misinterpreted.
5. Avoid asking probing questions that may recall prior circumstances. (Play can be a therapeutic method of ventilating feelings.)
6. Demonstrate acceptance of the child through physical affection and verbal kindness.
7. Recognize behaviors the child uses to gain attention or to display dissatisfaction with an unmet need; use positive reinforcement of the desirable behavior (the behavior may need to be modeled).
8. Praise the child's accomplishments to improve his self-esteem.
9. If the child is to return to the parent's care, integrate the parents into the daily routine; provide close supervision.

Medical diagnosis

The medical diagnosis is based on:
• injury inconsistent with the child's history
• signs of abuse or neglect in children
• inappropriate reaction (exaggerated or absent) of the parent to an injury.

Medical treatment

Treatment includes:
• caring for the physical maltreatment (injury or neglect)
• reporting the events or indicators to an appropriate child protection agency.

4 Perioperative Care

Because hospitalization can be a fearful and stressful event for a child, all pediatric patients need to be properly prepared for the experience. Before admission and undergoing any hospital procedure, patients should receive adequate age-appropriate explanations based on their developmental level. Family members providing the child's support system also need to be included in explanations so that their shared knowledge will enhance the child's understanding. Formal preadmission orientation meetings are most desirable.

During the preadmission meeting, the child and family should become acquainted with the actual equipment, special care areas, and anticipated pattern of planned procedures. The child is encouraged to experience through play, puppet shows, tours, and individualized discussion those events which are unique to the hospital experience.

Child-life specialists, who provide opportunities for therapeutic play and help meet the emotional needs of caregivers, assist the nursing staff in the larger pediatric unit or specialty hospital. Essential to the child's overall development, play is considered the "work of the child." Through play, the child is encouraged to express his beliefs and fears, such as those associated with upcoming procedures. As the child develops an increased understanding of the procedures and treatment, he becomes more secure, less tense, and less apprehensive. By controlling his behavior, the child improves his self-concept and general well-being.

☐ Preoperative care

Psychological preparation for surgery is as equally important as physical preparation. In planning interventions appropriate to the unique needs of each pediatric patient, you'll need to consider the following information:
• the child's age and developmental level
• the child's previous experiences with health care
• the family's role and value as a support system
• the implications of the operative procedure.

Because the strangeness of the operating room and associated areas generates fear in all age-groups, the pediatric patient should become as familiar as possible with the places and events associated with the surgical procedure before the actual experience. Children's picture books, videos, slide or tape presentations, and playroom models may be used to simulate real situations.

The most effective preprocedure intervention allows active participation of the pediatric patient and family. (Remember: In pediatric nursing, the patient *is* the family.) By manipulating equipment, visiting the preoperative holding area, operating room, and recovery room, and acting out or dressing up as members of the health care team, the child is better able to internalize upcoming experiences and events.

Nursing diagnosis

Anxiety related to fear of the unknown, separation from caregivers, lack of understanding of the purpose and outcome of procedures, and fear of mutilation, pain, or death (specify)

Desired outcome: The child experiences a reduction in anxiety as evidenced by relaxed facial expression and body language, verbalization of less fearfulness, and verbalization or acting out that reveals an understanding of anticipated events (as his developmental ability allows).

Interventions

Infants and young toddlers

1. Encourage the caregivers to stay with the child.
2. Orient the caregivers to the hospital environment, routines, and special procedures planned for the child.
3. Encourage the caregivers to verbalize fears so that clarification and increased understanding will minimize stress.
4. Allow the caregivers to remain with the child until anesthesia has occurred and to be at the crib side as the child responds after the event.
5. Use distraction to refocus the infant's or child's response after a stressful or painful event.
6. Provide consistency in assigning personnel to ensure continuity of care.

Mature toddlers and preschoolers

1. Use the interventions for the infants and young toddlers (listed above), if applicable.
2. Accept behaviors that indicate feelings of protest (such as resistance, physical aggression, and verbal uncooperativeness), saying, "I know this hurts; I feel bad too."
3. Accept regressive behaviors without comment.
4. Assess the child's preadmission preparation for hospitalization and procedures.
5. Plan experiences to allow the child and caregivers to gain further knowledge of anticipated events. For example, plan visits to special care areas, visits by members of the health care team (such as staff from the operating room or recovery room or an anesthesiologist), and play involving acting out and dressing up for procedures.
6. Schedule visits by a child-life specialist and time for therapeutic play.

7. Explain routine and special procedures and treatments before initiating them.

8. Avoid giving the child too much information at one time; allow adequate intervals to ensure he internalizes the knowledge. (A knowledge deficit may indicate the need for prehospitalization visits or early admission.)

9. Use descriptive words having less threatening meanings for the child. For example, use:
• "opening"—not "cutting"
• "drainage"—not "bleeding"
• "a special sleep from which you'll awaken after your operation"—not "being put to sleep" (may be associated with the death of a pet)
• "fix" the affected body part—not "remove" or "take away" (perceives removal of a body part as mutilation or a gaping hole or void in self).

10. Encourage caregivers to provide toys, photos, a security blanket, or a stuffed animal that may comfort the child.

11. Allow the child to wear his own clothing.

12. Prepare the child for the anticipated postoperative status. For example, explain that he may have:
• "hurts" (pain that may be relieved with medicine)
• bandages
• I.V. lines or other tubes
• casts or traction
• sutures. (Assure him that his moving about will not break the sutures; differentiate sutures from sewing stitches, which he may think are unreliable for holding seams together because they break or pull out.)

School-age children and adolescents

1. Use the interventions for the younger children (listed above), if applicable.

2. Assess the child's previous experiences and level of understanding before beginning preoperative teaching.

3. Encourage the expression of feelings; observe the child's body language and facial expression for evidence of fear and stress.

4. Acknowledge the child's fears and concerns.

5. Discuss anticipated events.

6. Reassure the child that his privacy will be respected.

Nursing diagnosis

Altered Health Maintenance related to change in usual nutritional elimination and sleep patterns

Desired outcome: Changes in the child's usual patterns are minimized as evidenced by maintenance of normal physiologic balance and prevention of infection.

Interventions

1. Limit the amount of time the child can have nothing by mouth

to a safe time frame, as determined by the anesthesiologist. For example, a child:
• under age 6 months should have no solids or milk for 8 hours before the anticipated time of surgery
• age 6 months to 3 years should have no solids or milk for 8 hours and no clear liquid for 6 hours before the anticipated time
• over age 3 should have no solids, milk, or clear liquid for 8 hours before the anticipated time.
2. Encourage the continent child to void and evacuate stool by providing privacy and, if possible, use of a toilet.
3. Plan nursing procedures and treatments at intervals that allow extended periods of undisturbed rest or sleep.
4. Keep noise and other environmental disturbances to a minimum.
5. Reduce the possibility of nosocomial infection by using caution in room assignments and careful asepsis among staff assigned to care for the child and by providing general physical cleanliness (preoperative bath).
6. Explain the reason for the postoperative routine of deep breathing, coughing, and range-of-motion exercises to all children who have the capacity to follow directions (perhaps as young as age 1).
7. Demonstrate and encourage return demonstrations of deep breathing and coughing.
8. Perform procedures and treatments as close as possible to the anticipated time; however, allow sufficient time for interruptions and unscheduled barriers.
9. Eliminate gaps between explanations and actions. (Preoperative medication should be given on time and with a brief description of its anticipated effect on the child's status, such as sleepiness or a dry mouth.)
10. Initiate intrusive or painful procedures, such as insertion of an I.V. line, catheterization, or nasogastric intubation, after an initial anesthetic has been administered, if possible. (An I.V. line may be used for administration of preoperative medication.)
11. Allow the child to maintain a maximum amount of control over events; give choices that provide an opportunity for him to cooperate with the health care team rather than submitting to their power or authority. (For example, ask if the child would like to go to the bathroom now or in 30 minutes. Or ask what kind of clear liquid he would like before not being allowed to drink.)

☐ Postoperative care

The child's status during the immediate postanesthesia period will depend, of course, on the surgical procedure. Generally, however, a child regaining consciousness will be restless and disoriented. Seeing and hearing familiar persons and objects will assist him during his recovery from anesthesia.

Keep in mind that postoperative pain, procedures, and new equipment may provoke fear that all is not well. The child will need to be reassured at this time that his status is normal. Hearing that he is doing fine will help relieve his anxiety and stress.

Nursing diagnosis

Ineffective Breathing Pattern related to depressant effects of anesthesia, medication, pain, anxiety, or positioning

Desired outcome: The child maintains his normal breathing pattern as evidenced by the rate, rhythm, and depth of respirations, the quality of breath sounds, and other signs indicative of an effective airway clearance.

Interventions

1. Monitor and report signs and symptoms of ineffective breathing or airway clearance, including shallow, slow respirations; hyperventilation; dyspnea; and retractions.
2. Monitor and report the child's blood gas levels.
3. Implement actions to decrease the child's fear and anxiety.
4. Use comfort measures, such as stroking, distraction, and administering sedatives and analgesics.
5. Administer analgesic medication in response to evidence of pain.
6. Assist the child with deep breathing, coughing, and range-of-motion exercises.
7. Change the child's position at least once every 2 hours; place him in Fowler's or semi-Fowler's position periodically, unless contraindicated.
8. Maintain adequate hydration to keep secretions liquefied.
9. Increase the child's activity, as allowed and tolerated.

Nursing diagnosis

Altered Comfort: Pain related to tissue trauma and reflex muscle spasm secondary to surgical procedure

Desired outcome: The child experiences diminished pain as evidenced by verbalization of greater comfort (when mature enough to communicate), relaxed facial expressions and body language, increased interest in the environment, and increased activity.

Interventions

1. Anticipate pain associated with the surgical procedure, especially in the nonverbal child.
2. Schedule pain medication instead of giving it as needed.
3. Observe the child for signs of discomfort, such as crying, irri-

tability, restlessness, poor response to feeding, body rigidity, and facial tenseness.

4. Observe the child for symptoms of discomfort, such as elevated vital signs, flushing or pallor, and diaphoresis.

5. Use comfort measures for pain relief, such as changing the child's position, supporting a body part, quiet conversation, stroking (for the younger child), distraction, or diversional activities.

6. Minimize activities that seem to aggravate pain; gently turn and reposition the child, and avoid confusion and disruption in the environment.

7. Assist with supporting the child's chest or abdominal incision by splinting, using a firmly placed pillow when the child deep-breathes and coughs.

8. Encourage the verbal child to express feelings.

5 Pediatric Resuscitation

Because an emergency can occur at any time in the clinical setting, cardiopulmonary resuscitation (CPR) training is prerequisite to any clinical experience. The information outlined below is not intended to replace that instruction. Rather, it serves a quick review to refresh your memory on pediatric variations. Before you're assigned to the pediatric unit, evaluate your knowledge about CPR; don't wait for an emergency to happen.

During orientation, be certain to learn where the crash cart or other emergency equipment is kept. Also, be sure to memorize the special code number used by health care workers when calling for help (most hospitals have their own special number). In all of the following emergencies, call for help with your assessment of a situation requiring resuscitation.

Keep in mind that, when giving CPR, age definitions are based on the following criteria:
• Infants: birth to age 1
• Children: age 1 to 8
• Adults: over age 8.

☐ Infant emergencies

Use the following interventions when administering emergency treatment to an infant. Remember that the most common cause of airway obstruction in infancy involves regurgitation and aspiration of feedings.

Treatment for choking

Determine whether the infant is conscious or unconscious, then follow the appropriate interventions as listed below:

Conscious infant

1. Assess for airway obstruction.
2. Give four back blows. To do so, place the infant over your forearm, along your thigh. Support the infant's head, face down, so that the head is lower than the trunk. Use the heel of your hand to deliver four back blows between the shoulder blades.
3. Give four chest thrusts. Sandwich the infant between your hands as above, turning him onto his back. Using two fingers placed vertically on the sternum, one fingerwidth below an imaginary line between the nipples, compress the chest four times.
4. Repeat these steps until the airway is cleared or the infant becomes unconscious.

Unconscious infant

1. Check for the presence of a foreign body. Placing your thumb in the infant's mouth over his tongue with your fingers under the jaw, lift upward. If you see a foreign body, remove it. (*Note:* Never attempt to remove a foreign body if you cannot see it.)
2. Attempt ventilation. Perform a head-tilt, chin-lift maneuver. (*Note:* Do not hyperextend the infant's neck.) Seal the infant's mouth and nose with your mouth and try to ventilate.
3. Give four back blows, as for a conscious infant.
4. Give four chest thrusts, as for a conscious infant.
5. Repeat steps 1 through 4 until you succeed in dislodging the foreign body or other medical help arrives.

Note: If you are uncertain that the unconscious infant is choking, reposition his head after the first unsuccessful ventilation attempt and try again. If the airway remains obstructed, proceed with the above cycle beginning at step 3. *Never* push on or into an infant's stomach, whether the infant is conscious or unconscious.

Infant CPR

Take the following steps when giving the infant CPR:

1. Assess for unresponsiveness.
2. Establish an airway. Place the infant on his back on a firm surface, keeping his head and neck supported. Tilt the infant's head and lift his chin to a "sniffing" position.
3. Assess for breathing by looking, listening, and feeling for breathlessness. If the infant is not breathing, ventilate twice, sealing the infant's nose and mouth with your mouth. Pause for deflation between ventilations.
4. Check for circulation by assessing for absence of a brachial pulse. If you cannot feel a pulse, perform five chest compressions (compressing downward ½" to 1" [1.3 to 2.5 cm]) with two or three fingers placed vertically on the infant's sternum, one finger-width below an imaginary line between the nipples.
5. Perform 10 cycles of one ventilation and five compressions (at a rate greater than 100 ventilations/minute).
6. Reassess the brachial pulse.
7. Resume the cycle of one ventilation and five compressions, pausing to assess the brachial pulse every few minutes. Continue this cycle until the infant responds or other medical help arrives.

☐ Child emergencies

Note the following when giving emergency treatment to a child:

Treatment for choking

Determine whether the child is conscious or unconscious, then proceed with the following interventions:

Conscious child

1. Assess the child's status and offer reassurance.
2. Perform the Heimlich maneuver, as for an adult.
3. Repeat the maneuver until you succeed in expelling the foreign body or the child becomes unconscious.

Unconscious child

1. Check for a foreign body. Open the child's mouth using a tongue-jaw lift maneuver. If you can see the foreign body, remove it. (*Note:* Never attempt to remove a foreign body if you cannot see it.)
2. Attempt ventilation. Perform a head-tilt, chin-lift maneuver, sealing the child's nose with your fingers and his mouth with yours.
3. Give abdominal thrusts (Heimlich maneuver). Kneeling at the child's feet, place one hand on top of the other at midpoint between the child's navel and xyphoid. Press inward and upward 6 to 10 times.
4. Repeat the above steps until you succeed in clearing the airway or other medical help arrives.
Note: If you're uncertain that the unconscious child is a choking victim, reposition the child's head and try again if the first ventilation attempt was unsuccessful. If the airway remains obstructed, proceed with the above cycle beginning at step 3.

Child CPR

Take the following steps when administering CPR to a child:
1. Assess for unresponsiveness.
2. Establish an airway. Place the child on his back on a firm surface, supporting his head and neck. Tilt the child's head, lifting his chin.
3. Assess for breathing by looking, listening, and feeling for breathlessness. If the child is not breathing, ventilate twice by pinching the child's nose with your fingers and sealing his mouth with yours. Pause for deflation between ventilations.
4. Check for circulation by assessing for a carotid pulse. If you cannot feel a pulse, perform five chest compressions (compressing downward 1" to 1½" [2.5 to 3.8 cm]) with the heel of one hand placed vertically on the sternum one fingerwidth above the xyphoid notch (avoid the xyphoid).
5. Perform 10 cycles of one ventilation and five compressions (at a rate of 80 to 100 ventilations/minute).
6. Reassess the child's status.
7. Resume cycles of one ventilation and five compressions, pausing to assess the carotid pulse every few minutes. Continue with this cycle until the child responds or other medical help arrives. (*Note:* If two rescuers are available to perform CPR, one will perform compressions, counting aloud and pausing after each five compressions to permit the other rescuer to ventilate.)

6 Psychosocial Aspects of Pediatric Care

Psychosocial factors play an important role in the care plan for any patient. However, the dependent state of the child, developmental ramifications, emotional overtones, family devastation, and parental guilt heighten the need for considering psychosocial needs in planning pediatric care.

Nursing diagnoses concerned with psychosocial needs are included in this section to avoid repeating the diagnoses within each disease or disorder. Nursing students are encouraged to refer to these diagnoses and to adapt them to individual child or family situations.

Nursing diagnosis
Fear related to the unfamiliar hospital environment, anticipated physical or psychological harm, and the possible threat of death
Desired outcome: The child or caregivers verbalize fears and demonstrate appropriate behaviors in dealing with them.

Interventions
1. Assess the existence and degree of fears by observing for trembling, tachycardia, elevated blood pressure, hyperventilation, aggressiveness, restlessness, diaphoresis, excessive verbalization, or questioning.
2. Evaluate contributing factors, such as communication of fear by the parent, age- or developmental-related fears, past experiences, knowledge deficit, or perception of the illness or hospitalization experience.
3. Reduce or eliminate contributing factors by making the environment familiar and comfortable, using the following measures:
• Implement home rituals and routines.
• Orient the child to the hospital in a calm, quiet, and simple manner.
• Encourage the caregivers to stay with the child.
• Make each day as predictable as possible (including consistent personnel).
• Provide a transitional object.
• Give explanations for all equipment and activities.
4. Discuss the child's fears with the caregivers by:
• explaining normal childhood fears
• assisting the caregivers in dealing with their own fears to prevent transmitting them to the child
• encouraging the caregivers to touch, hold, and stroke the child.
5. Use the following measures to provide outlets for expression of fears:
• Encourage the child or caregivers to verbalize fears.

• Use therapeutic play with the child.
• Accept the child's or caregivers' right to have fears, and work together on helping to solve them.
• Channel emotional energy into physical activity to dissipate fear (within limitations imposed by illness).
6. Provide the following information or referrals, as indicated:
• information on support groups
• knowledge about the illness and situation (can prevent fears from becoming anxieties with accompanying disequilibrium).

Nursing diagnosis

Ineffective Family Coping: Compromised or Disabled (or both) related to suffering or grief (or both) associated with the child's illness
Desired outcome: Caregivers identify strategies to cope with the child's illness.

Interventions

1. Assess the family's knowledge concerning the child's illness.
2. Provide information and correct misconceptions.
3. Identify resources available to help the family and child, such as parent support groups or existing local, state, or national agencies.
4. Acknowledge the effects of stress on the family, and assist with finding ways to alleviate it.
5. Encourage the family to participate in making and implementing plans. (Providing care will alleviate helpless feelings and ease the fear of transition to home management. Participation in planning will enhance self-esteem and provide a sense of control over the situation.)

Nursing diagnosis

Dysfunctional Family Grieving related to effects of the child's chronic or potentially fatal illness or to a sense of loss when the child is perceived as less than perfect
Desired outcome: The caregivers verbalize acceptance of the child's illness.

Interventions

1. Assess the family's current stage of grief.
2. Provide opportunities for verbalization.
3. Listen and acknowledge their right to grieve.
4. Be available to the family for listening or support.
5. Enlist the help of the family's significant others.
6. Recognize the need for professional counseling or clergy; offer referrals when appropriate.

Nursing diagnosis

Disturbance in Self-concept: Body Image, Self-esteem, or Personal Identity (specify) related to developmental crises coinci-

dental with illness or trauma
Desired outcome: The child verbalizes understanding and acceptance of self.

Interventions
1. Observe the child and listen for evidence of problems.
2. Establish rapport with the child.
3. Help the child recognize positive attributes.
4. Avoid reinforcement of poor body image by use of negative body language or facial expressions.
5. Observe caregiver interactions that may retard progress to the child's achieving a positive self-image.
6. Provide quality care to promote a good physiologic outcome of the disorder.
7. Discuss the need for, and possibility of, improvement through the use of a prosthesis, reconstructive surgery, make-up, or special clothing.
8. Spend time with the child; encourage the caregivers to spend time with the child to enhance the child's feelings of self-worth.

Nursing diagnosis
Powerlessness of the Child and Caregiver related to effects of illness and restrictions imposed by the hospital environment
Desired outcome: The child and caregivers make reasonable choices, assume control over aspects of care, and express optimism concerning the outcome of the illness.

Interventions
1. Orient the child and family to the hospital and personnel.
2. Assess the child's and family's knowledge of the situation.
3. Avoid imposing rules (when appropriate) just for the sake of adhering to rules.
4. Let the child and family know when acceptable choices are allowed.
5. Set attainable short-term goals, expanding on them as tolerated.
6. Openly discuss behaviors of helplessness.
7. Incorporate significant others into reinforcing the positive behaviors.
8. Provide opportunities for self-care within the limitations imposed by the disorder.
9. Accept requests and suggestions without criticism.
10. Provide opportunities to talk with children who have overcome similar illnesses.
11. Assist the family to participate in the child's care and to feel needed.

Nursing diagnosis
Altered Parenting related to an interrupted bonding process, ambivalence in feelings toward the ill child, or unrealistic expecta-

tions for the child's outcome
Desired outcome: The caregivers verbalize appropriate expectations for the child and demonstrate positive parenting behaviors.

Interventions
1. Identify cues of altered parenting, including negative verbalization by the caregivers, inattention to the child, delayed growth and development, obvious signs of abuse or neglect, and frequent abandonment to the care of others.
2. Assess the caregivers' parenting skills and available support systems.
3. Establish rapport with the caregivers by listening to their concerns.
4. Provide opportunities for bonding (may need to relax rules at times).
5. Encourage caregivers to meet their own needs.
6. Provide information on support groups, parenting classes, and community agencies; encourage participation.

Nursing diagnosis
Social Isolation (Self-imposed) related to illness and possibly accompanying depression
Desired outcome: The child expresses a desire to interact with others, seeks opportunities to participate in appropriate activities, and returns to school as soon as possible.

Interventions
1. Assess the child for depression.
2. Establish rapport with the child.
3. Determine which activities are within the child's present capabilities.
4. Formulate plans with the child and caregivers for establishing a daily schedule, including social activities.
5. Identify persons with similar interests.
6. Encourage peer visitation and telephone contacts.
7. Provide a stimulating environment, including positioning the child by a window with a view and providing a television.
8. Arrange for transportation to the children's play room and other areas where socialization may occur.
9. Don't force the child into socialization, but provide positive reinforcement of outreach efforts.
10. Formulate plans with the caregivers and school to prevent the child's falling below his grade or peer level.

Nursing diagnosis
Impaired Social Interaction related to limited physical mobility or therapeutic isolation
Desired outcome: The child verbalizes an understanding of the reasons for impaired socialization and interacts within the limits imposed.

Interventions

1. Use the interventions listed above in the previous diagnosis.
2. Explore the possibilities for activities and interaction.
3. Discourage invalidism imposed by self or caregivers.

Nursing diagnosis

Altered Family Process related to effects of the child's illness
Desired outcome: The family identifies problem-solving efforts to resolve the dysfunction-producing crisis.

Interventions

1. Establish a warm and caring atmosphere.
2. Assess family roles and patterns of communication.
3. Identify support systems and religious strengths.
4. Acknowledge the family's right to perceive their own problems.
5. Encourage communication within the family and with possible outside resources.
6. Avoid criticism.
7. Provide information, as needed.
8. Refer the family to support groups, counselors, clergy, or outside agencies, when needed.

Nursing diagnosis

Altered Growth or Development (or both): Delay or Regression related to effects of illness
Desired outcome: The child grows and functions appropriately for his age; caregivers participate with plans to assist the child in regaining or attaining developmental milestones.

Interventions

1. Assess and compare the child's growth and development status with that of norms.
2. Identify factors contributing to delay or regression.
3. Encourage the child to achieve a positive self-image.
4. Provide opportunities for self-care and independence, as his abilities permit.
5. Set realistic, short-term goals.
6. Identify educational and developmental resources in the community.

7 Medications

In any type of nursing specialty, medication administration is considererd a major nursing responsibility. However, in pediatric nursing, understanding mechanisms of action, calculating dosages, and evaluating therapeutic and adverse drug effects take on added significance.

Because a child's physical development can affect drug absorption and excretion, safe and effective dosages are based on factors other than size alone, such as the child's age and ability to metabolize drugs. For example, because of his immature liver and kidney function, a neonate may fail to metabolize some medications (such as sulfa drugs) and may excrete them unchanged. However, a child age 3 or older is capable of metabolizing some drugs at a faster rate (50% to 100% faster) than an adult because of his large hepatic surface area. For this reason, you may notice that pediatric dosages—usually expressed in terms of grams or milligrams per kilogram of body weight—are sometimes higher than adult dosages for specific medications. (*Note:* Some drugs used to treat adults and children have been known to have completely opposite effects when given to a child. The developing state of the child's neurochemistry may account for much of this variation.)

Checking dosages. Before administering any medication to a child, learn as much as you can about the drug and make sure the prescribed dosage falls within the recommended range for the child's age and weight. To check the dosage range, multiply the child's weight (in kilograms) by the safe dose factor or use one of the formulas listed below.

Clark's rule:
$$\frac{\text{Adult dose} \times \text{Child's weight (lb)}}{150} = \text{Dose}$$

Young's rule (for children over age 2):
$$\frac{\text{Adult dose} \times \text{Child's age (years)}}{\text{Child's age} + 12} = \text{Dose}$$

Fried's rule (for children under age 2):
$$\frac{\text{Adult dose} \times \text{Child's age (months)}}{150} = \text{Dose}$$

Body surface area (BSA) rule:
$$\frac{\text{Adult dose} \times \text{Child's body surface area (m}^2\text{)}}{1.7} = \text{Dose}$$

The BSA rule is perhaps the most accurate of the four rules mentioned. To determine the BSA, see *Calculating body surface area in children.*

Drug classifications. The following medications are arranged alphabetically by classification, according to their primary function in pediatrics. Each classification contains an alphabetical listing of generic drugs with pertinent information on each drug's dosage, route, uses, interactions, adverse effects, and nursing considerations.

Keep in mind that this is not intended as an exhaustive list of all pediatric medications, but rather as a quick reference of some of the most commonly used drugs in hospitalized children.

☐ Antibacterials and anti-infectives

Amoxicillin (Amoxil, Trimox), amoxicillin and clavulanate potassium (Augmentin)

Dosage
20 to 40 mg/kg/day in divided doses every 8 hours.

Route
P.O.

Uses
Treatment of respiratory, genitourinary, skin, or ear, nose, and throat infections.
Note: Amoxicillin-clavulanate combination provides increased resistance to beta-lactamase, an enzyme with the potential for inactivating penicillin.

Interactions
None significant.

Adverse reactions
Hypersensitivity reactions (do not give if allergic to penicillin); nausea, vomiting, and diarrhea.

Special considerations
• Drug may produce false-positive results on Clinitest.
• Drug may be taken without regard to food.

Ampicillin (Amcill, Omnipen, Principen)

Dosage
25 to 400 mg/kg/day in divided doses every 6 hours. Larger dosages may be given for meningitis infections.

Route
P.O., I.M., or I.V.

Uses
Treatment of gram-positive and -negative infections of the GI, genitourinary, and respiratory systems.

CALCULATING BODY SURFACE AREA IN CHILDREN

If the child's weight is proportional to his height, locate his weight and corresponding body surface area (BSA) in the boxed scale at left. Otherwise, use the nomogram on the right. Locate the child's height and weight on the scale, then connect the two measurements with a straight line. The point at which the line intersects the surface area column indicates the child's BSA.

For children of normal height and weight

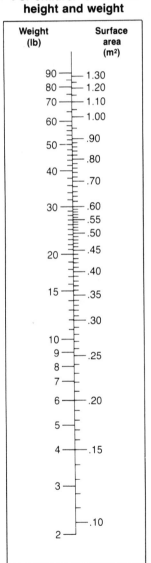

Nomogram

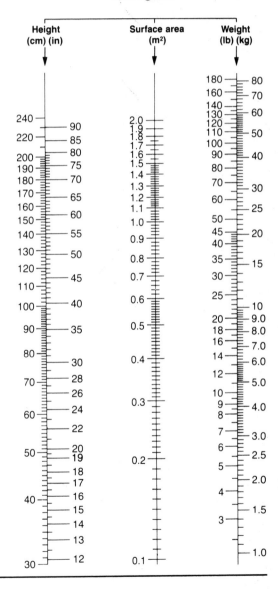

Interactions
None significant.

Adverse reactions
Hypersensitivity reactions (do not give if allergic to penicillin); nausea, vomiting, and diarrhea; possible overgrowth of *Candida*.

Special considerations
• "Ampicillin rash" commonly occurs 5 to 7 days after initiation of therapy, most often in children with Epstein-Barr virus.
• Drug must be taken on an empty stomach; absorption is decreased by citrus juices and various foods.

Cephalosporins (First generation: cefadroxil, cefazolin, cephalexin, cephalothin; second generation: cefaclor, cefoxitin, cefuroxime; third generation: cefotaxime, ceftazidime, ceftizoxime, ceftriaxone)

Dosage
See accompanying chart, *Cephalosporins*.

Route
See accompanying chart, *Cephalosporins*.

Uses
First generation: Treatment of skin and soft-tissue infections, pharyngitis, and urinary tract infections. Effective against gram-positive organisms, such as *Staphylococcus* and *Streptococcus*, and gram-negative organisms, such as *Escherichia coli* and *Hemophilus influenzae*.

Second generation: Treatment of otitis media, pneumonia, and soft-tissue infections. Provide good coverage of gram-positive, gram-negative, and beta-lactamase-producing organisms.

Third generation: Treatment of serious infections, including pneumonia, sepsis, and meningitis. Effective against gram-negative organisms, such as *E. coli, H. influenzae, Klebsiella, Neisseria, Proteus,* and *Psuedomonas*.

Interactions
None significant.

Adverse reactions
First generation
Cross-allergenicity to penicillin and other cephalosporins.
Second generation
Hypersensitivity reactions, especially in children sensitive to penicillin.
Third generation
Cross-allergenicity to penicillin and other cephalosporins; possible hypersensitivity, bleeding disorders, and pseudomembranous colitis.

Special considerations
Drug may be given with food.

CEPHALOSPORINS

Drug	Route	Dosage
FIRST GENERATION		
cefadroxil (Duricef)	P.O.	30 mg/kg/day every 12 hours
cefazolin (Ancef, Kefzol)	I.M. or I.V.	50 to 100 mg/kg/day every 8 hours
cephalexin (Keflex)	P.O.	25 to 50 mg/kg/day every 6 hours
cephalothin (Keflin)	I.M. or I.V.	75 to 125 mg/kg/day every 4 to 6 hours
SECOND GENERATION		
cefaclor (Ceclor)	P.O.	40 mg/kg/day every 8 hours
cefoxitin (Mefoxin)	I.M. or I.V	80 to 160 mg/kg/day every 4 to 6 hours
cefuroxime (Zinacef)	I.M. or I.V.	100 to 150 mg/kg/day every 8 hours
THIRD GENERATION		
cefotaxime (Claforan)	I.M. or I.V.	100 to 200 mg/kg/day every 6 to 8 hours
ceftazidime (Fortaz)	I.M. or I.V.	100 to 150 mg/kg/day every 8 hours
ceftizoxime (Cefizox)	I.M. or I.V.	150 to 200 mg/kg/day every 6 to 8 hours
ceftriaxone (Rocephin)	I.M. or I.V.	50 to 100 mg/kg/day every 12 to 24 hours

Chloramphenicol (Chloromycetin)

Dosage

For neonates, 25 to 50 mg/kg/day in divided doses every 6 hours. For other children, 50 to 100 mg/kg/day in divided doses every 6 hours.

Route

P.O. or I.V.

Uses

Treatment of life-threatening infections unresponsive to other drugs, such as *Salmonella typhi, Hemophilus influenzae,* meningitis, and rickettsia. Also used as part of the cystic fibrosis regimen.

Interactions

Chloramphenicol increases the effect of many drugs metabolized by the liver.

Adverse reactions

Serious and fatal blood dyscrasias; "gray baby" syndrome (in premature infants and neonates).

Special considerations

• Treatment requires hospitalization and frequent blood monitoring.

• This drug is not used to treat trivial infections.

• Extensive or repeated courses of therapy should be avoided.

• Serum levels must be monitored.

Co-trimoxazole (sulfamethoxazole-trimethoprim) (Bactrim, Septra)

Dosage

8 to 10 mg/kg/day every 12 hours for 10 days. May be given prophylactically 2 mg/kg/day in a single dose.

Route

P.O. or I.V.

Uses

Treatment of ampicillin-resistant urinary tract infections (UTIs), otitis media, shigellosis, or *Pneumocystis carinii* infections. May be used prophylactically (long-term in low dosages) for recurrent UTIs. Ineffective against streptococcal pharyngitis.

Interactions

• Co-trimoxazole may produce thrombocytopenia if given with thiazide diuretics.

• If given with warfarin, drug produces prolonged warfarin effect.

Adverse reactions

Nausea, vomiting, anorexia, rashes, and hives; possible Stevens-Johnson syndrome (a rare but extremely dangerous complication).

Special considerations

• Give adequate fluids to prevent crystalluria. Discontinue drug if rash occurs.

• Drug should not be given to children under age 2 months; kernicterus may result.

• Drug is contraindicated in children with impaired hepatic or renal function.

• Monitor liver and renal function tests.

Dicloxacillin sodium (Dynapen, Pathocil)

Dosage

12.5 mg/kg/day in four equal doses.

Route
P.O.

Uses
Treatment of penicillinase-producing strains of staphylococci.

Interactions
Dicloxacillin is antagonized by tetracycline.

Adverse reactions
Allergic reactions (do not give if allergic to penicillin).

Special considerations
• Medicinal taste may cause a problem with compliance.
• Other examples of penicillinase-resistant penicillins, including methicillin (Staphcillin), nafcillin (Unipen), and oxacillin (Prostaphlin), may be given I.M. or I.V.
• Drug is best absorbed on an empty stomach.

Erythromycin (E.E.S., E-Mycin, Eryc, EryPed, Erythrocin, Ilosone, Ilotycin)

Dosage
30 to 100 mg/kg/day in divided doses every 6 to 8 hours.

Route
P.O. or I.V.

Uses
Treatment of respiratory and skin infections of gram-positive cocci, chlamydial infection, and streptococcal pharyngitis when child is allergic to penicillin. Also used in the long-term prophylaxis of rheumatic fever.

Interactions
• Erythromycin is antagonized by clindamycin.
• Erythromycin increases theophylline levels; monitoring of theophylline levels is essential.
• Erythromycin produces increased carbamazepine levels if given concurrently.

Adverse reactions
GI upset, allergic reactions, and fungal infections.

Special considerations
• GI effects may be decreased by giving with food.
• Drug is absorbed well with food and may be given without regard to meals.

Erythromycin ethylsuccinate and sulfisoxazole acetyl (Pediazole)

Dosage
¼ teaspoon/kg/day in four doses.

Route
P.O.

Uses

Treatment of acute otitis media caused by *Hemophilus influenzae.*

Interactions

See "Erythromycin," page 239, and "Sulfisoxazole," page 242.

Adverse reactions

See "Erythromycin," page 239, and "Sulfisoxazole," page 242.

Special considerations

See "Erythromycin," page 239, and "Sulfisoxazole," page 242.

Neomycin sulfate (Mycifradin)

Dosage

40 to 100 mg/kg/day.

Route

P.O. and topical.

Uses

Reduction of intestinal ammonia production in Reye's syndrome. Also used in preoperative bowel preparation for bowel surgery.

Interactions

Neomycin may produce ototoxicity if given with loop diuretics and may cause respiratory failure if given with neuromuscular blocking agents.

Adverse reactions

Ototoxicity and nephrotoxocity.

Special considerations

• Keep the child well hydrated if therapy is prolonged.
• Assess neurologic status when drug is used to treat hepatic disorders.
• Similar aminoglycosides, including streptomycin, gentamicin, and tobramycin, also may cause ototoxicity or nephrotoxicity.

Oxytetracycline

See "Tetracycline," page 243.

Penicillin G benzathine, penicillin G potassium, penicillin G procaine, penicillin V potassium (Bicillin, Crysticillin, Pentids, Pen Vee K, Permapen, Wycillin)

Dosage

Varies with drug of choice.

Route

P.O., I.M., or I.V.

Uses

Treatment of gram-positive cocci, some gram-negative organisms, and spirochetes.

Interactions
None significant.

Adverse reactions
Allergic reactions.

Special considerations
• Always check for any known allergy to drug before administration.
• Watch for allergic reaction (particularly anaphylaxis) after administration, especially if given parenterally.
• If given P.O., drug is best given on an empty stomach.

Ribavirin (Virazole)

Dosage
The 6-g vial is reconstituted to 300 ml with sterile water to the recommended dilution of 20 mg/ml, then aerosolized for an average of 12 hours/day for 3 to 7 days.

Route
Aerosolized in a special aerosol unit and delivered via face mask, oxygen tent, or oxygen hood.

Uses
Treatment of infants and young children with severe lower respiratory tract infections caused by respiratory syncytial virus.

Interactions
No evaluation has been done on interaction with other drugs.

Adverse reactions
Respiratory deterioration associated with use in children with chronic obstructive lung disease or asthma; possible fetal harm (teratogenic in animals); possible cardiac arrest or hypertension; reticulocytosis, rash, and conjunctivitis.

Special considerations
• Ribavirin aerosol should not be used in infants requiring assisted ventilation; precipitation of the drug may interfere with safe and effective ventilation.
• Child should be hospitalized for this treatment.
• Standard supportive respiratory and fluid management should accompany ribavirin treatment with optimum monitoring of respiratory and fluid status.
• Drug is contraindicated in female patients who may become pregnant during or shortly after exposure to the drug. Pregnant staff must avoid exposure to this medication.
• Wearing of gloves is recommended when caring for these children. Some hospital protocols even require the use of masks and goggles.
• Drug should be mixed with only sterile (nonpreserved) water.
• Unused solution remaining in the aerosol unit should be discarded every 24 hours.

Rifampin (Rifadin, Rimactane)

Dosage
For the prophylactic treatment of *Hemophilus influenzae* meningitis, 20 mg/kg/day in a single dose for 4 days. To eliminate the carrier state of meningococcal meningitis, 10 mg/kg twice a day for 2 days.

Route
P.O.

Uses
Used effectively as a prophylactic agent against *H. influenzae* meningitis, and to eliminate the carrier state of meningococcal meningitis; also used as an antitubercular medication.

Interactions
Rifampin decreases the effectiveness of many drugs because of increased liver enzyme production.

Adverse reactions
Nausea, vomiting, diarrhea, abdominal pain, hemolytic anemia, and thrombocytopenia.

Special considerations
• Drug is best absorbed on an empty stomach. However, if child develops GI problems, capsules may be opened and mixed with applesauce.
• Drug may discolor body fluids (such as saliva, sweat, sputum, urine, and tears) orange and also may discolor contact lenses.
• Congenital anomalies may result if taken during pregnancy.

Sulfisoxazole (Gantrisin)

Dosage
Initially, 75 mg/kg/day, followed by a maintenance dosage of 150 mg/day in four doses.

Route
P.O., S.C., or I.V.

Interactions
Sulfisoxazole may produce cross-sensitivity if given with thiazide diuretics and oral hypoglycemic agents.

Adverse reactions
Allergic reactions, blood dyscrasias, crystalluria, and stone formation.

Special considerations
• Sulfonamides should not be given to children under age 2 months because of immature liver function, except to treat congenital toxoplasmosis.
• Various sulfa preparations and combinations also are available. Although dosages vary, adverse reactions and nursing considerations remain constant for all sulfa drugs.

Tetracycline hydrochloride (Achromycin, Cyclopar, Sumycin)

Dosage
15 to 25 mg/kg/day to a maximum of 250 mg/day in one to three doses.

Route
P.O., I.M., or I.V.

Uses
Treatment of severe acne, chlamydial infections, and various gram-positive and -negative infections. Also used as an alternative to penicillin to treat gonorrhea.

Interactions
• Tetracycline increases anticoagulant effects and antagonizes penicillin.
• Impaired absorption occurs if drug is given with antacids.

Adverse reactions
Photosensitivity; permanent discoloration of teeth in children under age 8.

Special considerations
• Do not use in children under age 8 unless other drugs are contraindicated.
• Oxytetracyclines, including doxycycline (Vibramycin) and oxytetracycline hydrochloride (Terramycin), have similar precautions and nursing considerations.
• Food and dairy products interfere with absorption.

☐ Anticonvulsants

Clonazepam (Klonopin)

Dosage
For children under age 10 or under 30 kg, 0.01 to 0.03 mg/kg/day (not to exceed 0.05 mg/kg/day), divided in two or three equal doses and given every 8 hours. Increase dosage by 0.25 to 0.5 mg every 3rd day to a maximum maintenance dosage of 0.1 to 0.2 mg/kg/day.

For children over age 10, 1.5 mg/day, divided in three doses and given every 8 hours. Increase dosage by 0.5 to 1 mg every 3 days, as needed. Maximum recommended daily dosage is 20 mg.

Route
P.O.

Uses
Treatment of absence-type seizures. Also used to treat akinetic and myoclonic seizures.

Interactions
None significant.

Adverse reactions
Blood dyscrasias, drowsiness, ataxia, behavioral disturbances,

diplopia, nystagmus, increased salivation, constipation, gastritis, appetite changes, abnormal thirst, sore gums, dysuria, enuresis, nocturia, urine retention, rash, and respiratory depression.

Special considerations
• Monitor for oversedation.
• Monitor complete blood count and liver function test results, as ordered.

Diazepam (Valium)

Dosage
For children under age 5, 0.2 to 0.5 mg every 2 to 5 minutes to a maximum of 5 mg. For children over age 5, 1 mg every 2 to 5 minutes to a maximum of 10 mg. May repeat dosages every 2 to 4 hours.

Route
I.V. or deep I.M.; I.V. route is more rapid and predictable.

Uses
Treatment of status epilepticus. Generally used as a sedative-hypnotic agent.

Interactions
• Diazepam potentiates the effects of other central nervous system (CNS) depressants.
• Use with cimetidine or valproic acid may increase CNS depression.

Adverse reactions
Hypotension (if given I.V.), respiratory depression, drowsiness, and lethargy.

Special considerations
• Assess cardiopulmonary status.
• Administer drug slowly to avoid respiratory or cardiac arrest.
• Do not mix with any other drug if giving I.V.
• For I.V. injections, use the largest vein possible and observe for signs of phlebitis.

Ethosuximide (Zarontin)

Dosage
For children age 3 to 6, 250 mg/day or 125 mg b.i.d.; may increase by 250 mg every 4 to 7 days up to 1.5 g daily. For children over age 6, 250 mg b.i.d. initially; may increase by 250 mg every 4 to 7 days up to 1.5 g daily.

Route
P.O.

Uses
Treatment of absence seizures.

Interactions
None significant.

Adverse reactions

Drowsiness, fatigue, dizziness, ataxia, irritability, euphoria, lethargy, myopia, hiccups, nausea, vomiting, diarrhea, gingival hypertrophy, weight loss, cramps, tongue swelling, anorexia, epigastric and abdominal pain, vaginal bleeding, urticaria, pruritic and erythematous rashes, hirsutism, lupus erythematosus–like symptoms, and blood dyscrasias.

Special considerations

• Monitor complete blood count every 3 months.
• When used alone in patients with mixed seizures, drug may increase frequency of generalized motor seizures.
• Drug may cause positive direct Coombs' test results.

Lorazepam (Ativan)

Dosage

0.04 mg/kg.

Route

I.V.

Uses

The treatment of choice for status epilepticus in many hospitals.

Interactions

Lorazepam potentiates the central nervous system effects of phenothiazines, narcotics, barbiturates, alcohol, antihistamines, monoamine oxidase (MAO) inhibitors, general anesthetics, and antidepressants.

Adverse reactions

Sedation and respiratory depression.

Special considerations

• Safe use of oral lorazepam in children under age 12 has not been established.
• Safe use of sublingual or parenteral lorazepam in children under age 18 has not been established.

Phenobarbital (Luminal)

Dosage

Loading dose is 3 to 5 mg/kg I.V.; may repeat every 10 to 15 minutes up to a total of 20 mg/kg. I.V. Injection rate should not exceed 60 mg/minute.

Maintenance dosage is 4 to 6 mg/kg P.O. daily, divided in two doses.

Route

I.V. and P.O.

Uses

Treatment of all forms of epilepsy.

Interactions

• Alcohol and other CNS depressants, including narcotic analgesics, cause excessive CNS depression.

• MAO inhibitors potentiate barbiturate effect.
• Rifampin causes decreased barbiturate levels.
• Primidone causes excessive phenobarbital blood levels.
• Valproic acid may cause increased phenobarbital levels.

Adverse reactions
Lethargy, headache, dizziness, nausea, vomiting, rash, urticaria, angioedema, and paradoxical excitability.

Special considerations
• Use I.V. injection for emergency treatment; administer slowly under close supervision. Monitor respirations and blood pressure.
• Assess for signs of barbiturate toxicosis, such as coma, asthmatic breathing, clammy skin, and hypotension. *Note:* Overdose can be fatal.

Phenytoin sodium (Dilantin)

Dosage
Loading dose is I.V. bolus of 15 mg/kg (not to exceed 50 mg/minute). Maintenance dosage is 4 to 8 mg/kg/day, P.O. or I.V., in one or two doses.

Route
I.V., P.O.

Uses
Treatment of generalized tonic-clonic and complex partial seizures; status epilepticus of the generalized tonic-clonic type; and nonepileptic seizures occurring after head trauma or Reye's syndrome.

Interactions
• Alcohol, folic acid, and loxapine succinate cause decreased phenytoin activity.
• Oral anticoagulants, antihistamines, chloramphenicol, diazepam, diazoxide, disulfiram, isoniazid, phenylbutazone, phenyramidol, salicylates, sulfamethizole, and valproate sodium cause increased phenytoin activity and toxicity.
• Tricyclic antidepressants in high doses may precipitate seizures, necessitating dosage adjustment.

Adverse reactions
Ataxia, slurred speech, confusion, dizziness, insomnia, nervousness, twitching, headache, gingivival hyperplasia, blood dyscrasias, hypotension, ventricular fibrillation, nystagmus, diplopia, blurred vision, vomiting, toxic hepatitis, measles or scarlet fever–like rash, exfoliative or purpuric dermatitis, lupus erythematosus–like symptoms, hirsutism, toxic epidermal necrolysis, periarteritis nodosa, lymphadenopathy, hyperglycemia, osteomalacia, and hypertrichosis.

Special considerations
• If administering drug parenterally, never use a cloudy solution.
• If giving direct I.V. push, flush tube with 5 ml of normal saline solution before and after drug administration. If unable to give direct I.V. push, mix with normal saline solution at a concentration of 100 mg/20 ml and administer over a 10-minute period using a separate I.V. administration set. Don't mix with dextrose 5% in water, because precipitation will occur. *Note:* Rapid I.V. push may cause cardiac dysrhythmias and arrest.
• Avoid giving phenytoin I.M., because drug may precipitate at injection site, causing necrosis and pain. Administration by this route also may result in erratic blood levels.
• Warn child and caregivers that drug may turn urine pink, red, or reddish brown.
• Stress the need for good oral hygiene and scheduling regular dental examinations to minimize the effects of gingival hyperplasia.
• Shake liquid suspension well before administration.
• Encourage caregivers to keep all follow-up appointments (usually every 4 to 6 weeks) to check for blood dyscrasias.

Valproic acid (Depakene)
Dosage
Initially, 15 mg/kg/day divided in two or three doses; may increase by 5 to 10 mg/kg/day at weekly intervals to a maximum of 30 mg/kg/day divided in two or three doses.

Route
P.O.

Uses
Long-term treatment of absence, myoclonic, and tonic-clonic seizures. It is also administered rectally for status epilepticus refractory to other anticonvulsants.

Interactions
Valproic acid may cause increased phenobarbital levels.

Adverse reactions
Inhibited platelet aggregation, thrombocytopenia, increased bleeding time, sedation, emotional upset, depression, psychosis, aggression, hyperactivity, behavioral deterioration, muscle weakness, tremor, nausea, vomiting, indigestion, diarrhea, abdominal cramps, constipation, increased appetite, weight gain, anorexia, pancreatitis, enzyme elevation, toxic hepatitis, and alopecia.

Special considerations
• Monitor liver function studies, platelet count, and prothrombin time before starting therapy and every 2 months afterward.
• If child develops tremors, reduce dosage, as ordered.
• To reduce GI adverse reactions and produce uniform blood

drug levels, give drug with food or milk.

• Drug may produce false-positive test results for ketones in urine.

• Drug is available as a palatable red syrup, which should be kept out of child's reach. *Note:* Because syrup is absorbed more rapidly, its peak effect occurs within 15 minutes.

• To avoid mouth and throat irritation, instruct child not to chew capsules. Also, don't mix syrup with carbonated beverages.

☐ Asthma medications

Albuterol (Proventil, Ventolin)

Dosage
0.1 mg/kg of syrup, up to 2 mg every 8 hours; or one or two puffs aerosol inhaler every 4 to 6 hours.

Route
P.O. or inhaled.

Uses
Treatment of bronchospasm in children with reversible obstructive airway disease. Also used to treat exercise-induced bronchospasm.

Interactions
See "Epinephrine."

Adverse reactions
See "Epinephrine."

Special considerations
• The aerosol form is used by some doctors in children under age 12 despite manufacturer's directions.

• Albuterol has less cardiac stimulation than epinephrine.

Aminophylline (Aminophyllin)

Dosage
For infants, $(0.3 \times$ child's age in months$) + 8$ equals the recommended dosage (mg/kg/day). For children age 1 to 9, 1 mg/kg/hour I.V. or 28 mg/kg/day P.O. For children age 10 to 16, 0.75 mg/kg/hour I.V. or 21 to 24 mg/kg/day P.O. For children over age 16, 0.5 mg/kg/hour I.V.

Route
I.V. or P.O.

Uses
Treatment of asthma and chronic obstructive pulmonary disease.

Interactions
See "Theophylline," page 251.

Adverse reactions
See "Theophylline," page 251.

Special considerations
See "Theophylline," page 251.

Cromolyn (Intal)

Dosage
Initially, 20 mg four times daily via nebulizer or spinhaler.

Route
Inhalant.

Uses
Used prophylactically for asthma attacks and as a mast cell stabilizer (inhibits the release of histamine). Especially effective as a prophylaxis for exercise-induced asthma.

Interactions
None significant.

Adverse reactions
Coughing, sneezing, and nausea.

Special considerations
• Avoid use in children under age 2.
• Drug is ineffective in treating acute asthmatic attacks.

Epinephrine (Adrenalin, Sus-Phrine)

Dosage
0.01 to 0.025 ml/kg S.C. in a 1:1,000 solution. May be given every 15 to 20 minutes, to a maximum of three doses, during an acute asthmatic attack or for anaphylaxis.

Sus-Phrine (epinephrine in suspension in a 1:200 solution) often is given after the initial dose (or first two doses) of epinephrine to provide both immediate and sustained effects. Dose is 0.005 ml/kg S.C. to a maximum of 0.15 ml; may repeat every 6 hours.

Route
S.C.

Uses
Used therapeutically as a bronchodilator and cardiac stimulant. Sustained action form (Sus-Phrine) provides sustained effects.

Interactions
• Epinephrine produces enhanced effect when used with decongestants.
• Hypertensive crisis is possible if given with MAO inhibitors.

Adverse reactions
Tremors, insomnia, tachycardia, and dysrhythmias.

Special considerations
• Verify dosage with the supervisory nurse before administration.

• Monitor the child's pulse and respiratory rates and blood pressure.
• Assess lung sounds for effective relief of respiratory distress.
• Avoid I.M. administration.

Isoetharine (Bronkosol)

Dosage
Depends on solution strength.

Route
Aerosol or hand-held nebulizer.

Uses
Treatment of bronchial asthma and reversible bronchospasm that may occur with bronchitis or emphysema.

Interactions
See "Epinephrine," page 249.

Adverse reactions
See "Epinephrine," page 249.

Special considerations
See "Albuterol," page 248.

Metaproterenol sulfate (Alupent, Metaprel)

Dosage
1.3 to 2.6 mg/kg/day P.O. in three doses. Alternatively, two or three puffs of a metered-dose inhaler (0.65 mg/puff) every 4 to 6 hours to a maximum of 12 puffs daily. Also may be given by hand-held nebulizer as an inhalant solution (a 5% solution of 0.3 ml dissolved in 3 ml of normal saline solution) every 4 to 6 hours, as needed.

Route
P.O. or inhalation.

Uses
Used as a bronchodilator.

Interactions
See "Epinephrine," page 249.

Adverse reactions
See "Epinephrine," page 249.

Special considerations
Many doctors use metaproterenol in children under 12 despite manufacturer's directions.

Steroids (beclomethasone dipropionate, hydrocortisone sodium succinate, methylprednisolone sodium succinate, prednisone)

Dosage
• Beclomethasone dipropionate (Vanceril): Not recommended for children under age 6. For children age 6 to 12, one or two puffs

of a metered-dose inhaler every 6 to 8 hours. For children over age 12, two puffs every 6 to 8 hours.
• Hydrocortisone sodium succinate (Solu-Cortef): 10 to 20 mg/kg/day I.V. or I.M.
• Methylprednisolone sodium succinate (Solu-Medrol): 0.4 to 2 mg/kg/day I.V. or I.M.
• Prednisone (Deltasone): 1 to 2 mg/kg/day P.O.

Route
I.V., I.M., P.O., or inhalation.

Uses
Used as an anti-inflammatory and to produce increased sensitivity to beta-adrenergics.

Interactions
• Steroids may cause increased hyperkalemia when used with some diuretics.
• Phenytoin and phenobarbital decrease steroidal effect.

Adverse reactions
Cushingoid appearance, cataracts, stunted growth, osteoporosis, and decreased resistance to infection. Inhaler also may cause oral or pharyngeal candidiasis.

Special considerations
• Dosage will be tapered when discontinuing corticosteroid therapy.
• Long-term use is avoided because of numerous possible adverse effects.
• Adrenal insufficiency may result from long-term corticosteroid therapy because of diminished pituitary stimulation.

Theophylline (Elixophyllin, Slo-bid, Slo-Phyllin, Somophyllin, Theobid, Theo-Dur, Theophyl)

Dosage
Ideally, dosages are based on serum theophylline levels. However, if unavailable, maximum dosages are as follows:
• Children age 1 to 9: 24 mg/kg/day P.O. or 0.8 mg/kg/hour I.V.
• Children age 10 to 12: 20 mg/kg/day P.O. or 0.6 mg/kg/hour I.V.
• Children age 13 to 16: 18 mg/kg/day P.O.
• Children over age 16: 0.4 mg/kg/hour I.V.

Route
P.O. or I.V.

Uses
Used to manage acute and chronic asthma.

Interactions
• Smoking (active or passive) decreases theophylline levels.
• Erythromycin, clindamycin, and cimetidine produce decreased

clearance, possibly resulting in toxic serum levels.
• High-protein diet decreases theophylline's half-life.
• High-carbohydrate diet increases theophylline's half-life.

Adverse reactions
Headache, nausea, vomiting, insomnia, agitation, restlessness,
tachycardia, palpitations, muscle twitching, and possible seizures.

Special considerations
• Once administered, theophylline is the active form of amino-
phylline.
• Use with extreme caution (if at all) in patients with cardiac or
hepatic disease.
• Make sure all I.V. preparations are hung by a supervisory nurse
after double-checking dosage with a second nurse.
• Monitor and record baseline vital signs and lung sounds before
starting medication and every 2 hours while infusing.
• Make sure sustained-release tablets are taken whole and are not
chewed or crushed.
• Capsules and gyrocaps may be opened and given with food.

☐ Cardiac medications

Atropine sulfate
Dosage
0.01 to 0.03 mg/kg I.V. bolus.

Route
I.V.

Uses
Treatment of sinus bradycardia and heart block.

Interactions
• Atropine may impair absorption of other drugs.
• Additive effect may occur if given with antihistamines or tri-
cyclic antidepressants.

Adverse reactions
Tachycardia, increased respirations, restlessness, irritability, disorientation, depression, urine retention, thirst, headache, constipation, flushing, and warm, dry skin.

Special considerations
• Monitor heart rate and rhythm to determine drug effects.
• Watch for and report signs of drug toxicity.
• Store drug in a light-resistant container.

Digoxin (Lanoxin)
Dosage
For premature infants and newborns, 25 to 40 mcg/kg/day I.V.
bolus in three divided doses. Maintenance dosage is 20% to 30%

of total loading dose divided in two equal parts and given 12 hours apart.

For children under age 2, 60 to 80 mcg/kg/day P.O. in three equal doses. Maintenance dosage is 20 to 25 mcg/kg/day in two equal doses given 12 hours apart.

For children age 2 and older, 40 to 60 mcg/kg/day P.O. or 20 to 40 mcg/kg/day I.V. For either route, give ½ of dosage immediately, then ¼ of dosage every 8 hours for two doses. Maintenance dosage is 10 to 15 mcg/kg/day P.O. (or 8 to 12 mcg/kg/day I.V.) divided in two equal doses and given every 12 hours.

Uses
Treatment of CHF, atrial fibrillation or flutter, paroxysmal atrial tachycardia, and supraventricular tachydysrhythmias.

Interactions
• If given with antacids, decreased absorption occurs.
• Toxicity may occur if given with any medication that decreases potassium levels (such as diuretics and some antibiotics).

Adverse reactions
Changes in heart rate and rhythm, irritability of heart muscles and conduction system, anorexia, nausea, vomiting, excessive salivation, abdominal pain, diarrhea, headache, fatigue, general malaise, disorientation, visual disturbances, and skin reactions (such as pruritus, urticaria, and facial edema).

Special considerations
• Monitor apical pulses for 1 minute. Withhold drug and notify doctor if apical pulse rate is less than 90 beats/minute or is outside of specified parameters.
• Monitor patients with digitalis toxicity for dysrhythmias.
• Monitor fluid intake and output.
• Watch for signs of hypokalemia; monitor serum potassium levels.
• Observe for the following positive responses to drug: improved heart rate and rhythm, improved respirations, weight reduction, and diuresis.

Dobutamine hydrochloride (Dobutrex)

Dosage
2.5 to 15 mcg/kg/minute I.V. Dilute reconstituted solution in at least 250 ml of dextrose 5% in water or normal saline solution. Adjust rate according to response.

Route
I.V.

Uses
Used for short-term parenteral therapy to strengthen heart muscle contractions (inotropic effect) and to treat heart failure caused by organic heart disease or heart surgery.

Interactions
• Hypertension or dysrhythmias may occur if given with MAO inhibitors or tricyclic antidepressants.
• Dobutamine may be ineffective if given with beta blockers.

Adverse reactions
Increased heart rate, blood pressure, and ectopic ventricular beats; although rare, may cause nausea, headache, chest pain, and shortness of breath.

Special considerations
• Correct hypovolemia, if possible, before giving drug.
• Continuously monitor blood pressure and heart rate.
• Do not give drug with an alkaline solution.
• Do not administer sodium bicarbonate through an I.V. line containing dobutamine.
• Use solutions containing dobutamine within 24 hours. *Note:* Although solutions may be discolored, potency of drug is unaffected.

Dopamine hydrochloride (Intropin)

Dosage
2 to 20 mcg/kg/minute; may be increased to no more than 20 mcg/kg/minute.

Route
I.V.

Uses
Treatment of cardiogenic shock. Also used to treat hypovolemic shock associated with trauma, septicemia, open heart surgery, renal failure, and CHF.

Interactions
• Dopamine reacts with I.V. phenytoin to produce severe bradycardia and decreased blood pressure.
• Reduced effectiveness occurs if given with beta blockers.

Adverse reactions
Cardiac dysrhythmias, palpitations, widening of QRS complexes, headache, dizziness, pallor, diaphoresis, nausea, vomiting, restlessness, tremors, weakness, respiratory difficulty, angina-like pain, and hypotension.

Special considerations
• Monitor cardiac conduction continuously, blood pressure every 5 minutes, and urine output every hour. Notify doctor of any changes.
• Check the infusion site frequently for extravasation. If extravasation occurs, notify doctor, who may infiltrate the site using 5 to 10 mg of phentolamine hydrochloride with 10 to 15 ml of normal saline solution.
• Administer drug by infusion pump.

• Mix drug with I.V. solution just before administration.
• Do not mix dopamine with other drugs.

Epinephrine hydrochloride (Adrenalin Chloride)

Dosage
0.1 to 1 mcg/kg/minute as a 1:50,000 solution. Regulate rate by response.

Route
I.V.

Uses
Treatment of cardiac and circulatory failure, hypotensive states, allergic reactions (including anaphylactic shock), angioneurotic edema, and status asthmaticus.

Interactions
• Increased effect occurs if given with decongestants.
• Hypertensive crisis may occur if given with MAO inhibitors.

Adverse reactions
Cerebral hemorrhage, cardiac dysrhythmias, palpitations, widened pulse pressure, precordial pain, headache, nervousness, vertigo, tremors, diaphoresis, nausea, weakness, dizziness, and tachycardia.

Special considerations
• Do not expose drug to light, heat, or air.
• When preparing to give drug I.V., first take the patient's blood pressure and pulse rate. Then, after initiating therapy, closely monitor the patient every minute until desired effect is achieved; then, monitor every 2 minutes until the patient stabilizes. After he stabilizes, monitor blood pressure every 15 minutes.
• If patient has a sharp increase in blood pressure, give rapid-acting vasodilators, as ordered.

Isoproterenol hydrochloride (Isuprel)

Dosage
1 mg in 100 ml of dextrose 5% in water infused at a rate of 0.1 to 0.5 mcg/kg/minute. Adjust rate to patient response.

Route
I.V.

Uses
Treatment of cardiac standstill, Stokes-Adams and carotid sinus syndromes, bradycardia, and atrioventricular (AV) heart block.

Interactions
• Hypertensive crisis may occur if given with MAO inhibitors.
• Diminished effectiveness occurs if given with beta blockers.

Adverse reactions
Tachycardia, palpitations, bronchial edema, flushing, headache,

dysrhythmias, chest pain, tremors, anxiety, fatigue, nausea, and vomiting.

Special considerations
• Closely monitor the patient's heart rate and rhythm, central venous and arterial pressures, arterial blood gas (ABG) levels, and urine output. If heart rate exceeds 130 beats/minute, slow down or discontinue drug.
• Administer drug with an infusion pump.

Lidocaine hydrochloride (Xylocaine)

Dosage
1 mg/kg I.V. bolus; may be repeated, but not to exceed 3 mg/kg/day. Alternatively, 1 g in 250 ml dextrose 5% in water infused at a rate of 20 to 40 mcg/kg/minute.

Route
I.V.

Uses
Treatment of ventricular tachycardia and acute ventricular dysrhythmias.

Interactions
• Toxicity may occur if given with beta blockers, phenytoin, or quinidine.
• Decreased metabolism if given with cimetidine.

Adverse reactions
Dizziness, restlessness, apprehension, tinnitus, visual disturbances, hearing loss, vomiting, difficulty breathing or swallowing, twitching, tremors, convulsions, hypotension, cardiovascular collapse, cardiac conduction disorders, bradycardia, cardiac and respiratory arrest, and numbness in extremities, lips, or tongue.

Special considerations
• Monitor heart rate and rhythm and blood pressure during administration.
• Observe for adverse reactions; notify the doctor if any occur.
• If symptoms of toxicity, such as dizziness, appear, stop infusion immediately. *Note:* Continued infusion could lead to convulsions and coma.
• When administering drug by I.V. infusion, use an infusion pump.
• During antiarrhythmic therapy, never use lidocaine with epinephrine added.

Propranolol hydrochloride (Inderal)

Dosage
0.01 to 0.15 mg/kg I.V. bolus, given slowly. Dose may be repeated every 6 to 8 hours.

Route
I.V.

Uses
Treatment of supraventricular, atrial, and ventricular dysrhythmias. Also used to treat hypertension and angina.

Interactions
• Increased effects occur if given with cimetidine.
• Propranolol potentiates digitalis effects and the effects of other antihypertensives.
• Decreased effectiveness of some bronchodilators (such as epinephrine) may occur.

Adverse reactions
CHF or circulatory collapse, hypotension, cardiac disturbances (including bradycardia, angina, and asystole), AV heart block, GI disturbances, CNS disturbances (including hallucinations, syncope, uncoordinated movements, dizziness, insomnia, confusion, and depression), rashes, peripheral vascular insufficiency, bronchospasms, wheezing, and blood sugar abnormalities.

Special considerations
• Monitor apical pulse rate before and after administration. If pulse rate is below 50 beats/minute, withhold drug and notify doctor.
• Auscultate the patient's lungs for crackles and his heart for gallop rhythm during administration. If found, notify doctor.
• Keep atropine sulfate on hand to counteract possible bradycardia.
• Observe diabetic patients for insulin shock. (Propranolol masks characteristic signs of hypoglycemia, including tachycardia and diaphoresis.)
• When stopping therapy, gradually slow infusion rate.

Sodium bicarbonate

Dosage
For cardiac arrest, give 2 to 4 mEq/kg I.V. bolus. Subsequent doses are based on ABG measurements to a maximum of 8 mEq/kg/day.

Route
I.V.

Uses
Used for cardiac arrest and to treat metabolic acidosis.

Interactions
Oral form interferes with absorption of other orally administered drugs.

Adverse reactions
GI disturbances (such as abdominal cramps, anorexia, nausea, and vomiting), dizziness, convulsions, thirst, and diminished respirations; with overdose: alkalosis, hypernatremia, and hyperosmolarity.

Special considerations
• Drug may be added to I.V. solution unless solution contains epinephrine or norepinephrine.
• Do not infuse through an I.V. line containing lactated Ringer's solution (or any other solution containing calcium) or the drug will precipitate.
• Obtain ABG and serum electrolyte measurements during administration, and report any changes.
• Sodium bicarbonate may cause tissue sloughing if extravasation occurs.

Verapamil hydrochloride (Calan, Isoptin)

Dosage
For children under age 1, 0.1 to 0.2 mg/kg I.V. bolus; repeat dose in 30 minutes. For children age 1 to 15, 0.1 to 0.3 mg/kg I.V. bolus; repeat dose in 30 minutes. Not to exceed 10 mg per single dose. *Note:* Administer all I.V. bolus doses over at least 2 minutes.

Route
I.V.

Interactions
• Verapamil produces enhanced digitalis effect and beta-blocker activity.
• Decreased effectiveness occurs if given with phenytoin.

Adverse reactions
Brief hypotension (usually transient and asymptomatic), bradycardia (including AV blocks), and paradoxical increase in ventricular rate in atrial fibrillation or atrial flutter.

Special considerations
• Monitor blood pressure for signs of hypotension. Patient may complain of headache or dizziness.
• Monitor heart rate frequently.
• Do not administer beta-adrenergic drugs I.V. within 4 hours after giving verapamil. These drugs depress myocardial activity and slow AV conduction.

☐ Chemotherapeutic medications

Asparaginase (Elspar)

Dosage
Dosage regimens are complicated and varied. When used without other agents, the recommended dosage is 200 IU/kg/day for 28 days.

Route
I.V. or I.M.

Uses
Treatment of leukemia.

Interactions
Asparaginase abolishes methotrexate effect.

Adverse reactions
Allergic reactions (including anaphylactic shock), fever, nausea, vomiting, and weight loss; toxic effects: liver dysfunction, hyperglycemia, and renal failure.

Special considerations
• Keep epinephrine (1:1,000) at the patient's bedside. Usual dose is 0.01 mg/kg.
• Record signs of allergic reaction, such as urticaria, facial edema, hypotension, or abdominal cramps.
• Check the patient's weight daily.
• Normally, BUN and ammonia levels increase as a result of drug use; such increases do not indicate liver damage.
• Check the patient's urine for sugar content.

Bleomycin sulfate (Blenoxane)

Dosage
0.25 to 0.50 units/kg once or twice per week.

Route
I.V., I.M., S.C.

Uses
Treatment of Hodgkin's lymphoma.

Interactions
Pulmonary toxicity may occur if given at lower doses when used with other antineoplastic agents.

Adverse reactions
Allergic reaction (including fever, chills, hypotension, and anaphylaxis), nausea, vomiting, stomatitis, and cumulative effects (including rash, hyperpigmentation, skin thickening, ulceration, skin peeling, nail changes, alopecia, and pneumonitis with infiltrate that can progress to fatal fibrosis).

Special considerations
• Give a test dose before administering therapy.
• Keep diphenhydramine hydrochloride and epinephrine at the patient's bedside.
• Hypersensitivity usually occurs with initial one or two doses.
• Concentration of drug in skin and lungs accounts for toxic effects.

Carmustine (BiCNU)

Dosage
200 mg/m² every 6 weeks.

Route
I.V.

Uses
Treatment of Hodgkin's and other lymphomas, brain tumors, and neuroblastomas.

Interactions
None known.

Adverse reactions
Nausea and vomiting (usually within 2 to 6 hours), bone marrow depression (4 to 6 weeks later), burning pain along I.V. infusion site, and flushing and facial burning on infusion.

Special considerations
• Use drug cautiously if bone marrow depression is already present.
• Avoid extravasation; contact with skin causes brown spots.
• Drug crosses blood-brain barrier.

Chlorambucil (Leukeran)

Dosage
0.1 to 0.2 mg/kg/day for 3 to 6 weeks (typically, 4 to 10 mg/day for an average patient).

Route
P.O.

Uses
Treatment of Hodgkin's disease and chronic lymphocytic leukemia.

Interactions
None known.

Adverse reactions
Nausea, vomiting, bone marrow depression, diarrhea, dermatitis, and (rarely) hepatotoxicity.

Special considerations
• Drug usually has a slow onset of action.
• Adverse reactions usually are related to high doses.

Cisplatin (Platinol)

Dosage
Dosage varies according to the specific type of cancer being treated as well as the chemotherapy protocols in which combinations are used.

Route
I.V.

Uses
Treatment of testicular and ovarian carcinomas, osteogenic sarcomas, and neuroblastomas.

Interactions
Drug is effective when used in combination with bleomycin and vinblastine.

Adverse reactions
Renal toxicity (usually severe), nausea and vomiting (usually severe, occurring within 1 to 4 hours), bone marrow depression (usually mild, occurring 2 to 3 weeks later), ototoxicity, neurotoxicity (similar to that of vincristine), and anaphylactic reactions.

Special considerations
• Assess renal function before giving drug.
• Maintain hydration before and during therapy. (Urine specific gravity may be used to assess hydration.)
• Monitor intake and output.
• Administer an antiemetic, usually chlorpromazine, with therapy.
• Advise the child and caregivers about the possibility of ototoxicity; alert them to specific signs and symptoms to report.
• Observe for signs of allergic reaction.
• Keep oxygen, suction equipment, and emergency drugs on hand at the patient's bedside.

Corticosteroids (prednisone)
Various other corticosteroids are used; however, prednisone is commonly selected.

Dosage
Dosage varies with chemotherapy protocol. Commonly, dosage is 40 mg/m²/day in three doses for 28 days, then tapered.

Route
P.O.; also I.V. or I.M. (rarely used).

Uses
Treatment of leukemia and Hodgkin's and other lymphomas.

Interactions
Hypokalemia may occur if used with diuretics and penicillins.

Adverse reactions
• With short-term use: mild bone marrow depression, moon face, fluid retention, weight gain, euphoria, increased appetite, gastric irritation, and susceptibility to infection.
• With long-term use: mood changes, hirsutism, trunk obesity (buffalo hump), thinned extremities, muscle wasting and weakness, osteoporosis, poor wound healing, bruising, potassium loss, gastric bleeding, hypertension, and diabetes mellitus.

Special considerations
• Explain to the child and caregivers the expected effects of therapy, especially in terms of body image, increased appetite, and personality changes.
• Monitor weight gain; evaluate true weight (muscle mass) from water retention.
• Recommend a low-sodium diet, if needed.
• Administer drug with an antacid early in the morning (sometimes given every other day to minimize effects).

• Give drug with food, if needed, to disguise bitter taste.
• Observe potential infection sites; usual inflammatory response and fever may be absent with infection.
• Encourage the child to eat foods high in potassium (such as bananas, raisins, prunes, coffee, and chocolate).
• Test stools for occult blood.
• Test urine for sugar and acetone.

Cyclophosphamide (Cytoxan)

Dosage
Loading dose is 40 to 50 mg/kg/day I.V. for 2 to 5 days, or 1 to 5 mg/kg/day P.O. Maintenance dosage varies: 1 to 5 mg/kg/day P.O.; 10 to 15 mg/kg/day I.V. for 7 to 10 days; or 3 to 5 mg/kg/day twice weekly.

Route
P.O., I.V., I.M., intraperitoneal, intrapleural, or intrathecal.

Uses
Treatment of leukemia, Hodgkin's and other lymphomas, neuroblastomas, retinoblastomas, and sarcomas.

Interactions
Rate of metabolism and leukopenic activity are potentiated by chronic administration of high doses of phenobarbital.

Adverse reactions
Nausea and vomiting (usually within 3 to 4 hours), bone marrow depression (7 to 14 days later), alopecia, hemorrhagic cystitis, severe immunosuppression, mucosal ulceration, hyperpigmentation, transverse ridging of nails, and infertility.

Special considerations
• Bone marrow depression has platelet-sparing effect.
• Force fluids before administering drug and for 2 days afterward to prevent chemically induced cystitis. Also, encourage frequent voiding, even during the night.
• Warn child and caregivers to report burning on urination or hematuria immediately to the doctor.

Dactinomycin (Cosmegen)

Dosage
15 mcg/kg/day for 5 days repeated every 2 to 4 weeks.

Route
I.V.

Uses
Treatment of Wilms' tumor, neuroblastomas, and sarcomas.

Interactions
Enhanced bone marrow depression occurs if given with other chemotherapeutic agents.

Adverse reactions

Nausea and vomiting (2 hours after administration), bone marrow depression (especially platelet), immunosuppression, mucosal ulceration, diarrhea, anorexia (may last a few weeks), alopecia, acne, erythema or hyperpigmentation of previously irradiated skin, fever, and malaise.

Special considerations

• Extravasation causes skin necrosis and pain; administer drug through a free-flowing infusion.
• Drug enhances cytotoxic effects of radiation but increases toxic effects.
• Use of drug may cause desquamation of irradiated tissue.

Daunorubicin hydrochloride (Cerubidine)

Dosage

As a single agent: 60 mg/m^2/day on days 1, 2, and 3 every 3 to 4 weeks. If used in combination with other chemotherapeutic agents, dosage is reduced to 45 mg/m^2/day on days 1, 2, and 3 of first course, then 45 mg/m^2/day on days 1 and 2 of second course (usually in 3 to 4 weeks). Dosage modification may be required based on serum bilirubin and creatinine levels if hepatic or renal impairment exists.

Route

I.V.

Uses

Treatment of acute myeloblastic leukemia.

Interactions

None known.

Adverse reactions

See "Doxorubicin."

Special considerations

See "Doxorubicin."

Doxorubicin hydrochloride (Adriamycin RDF)

Dosage

60 to 75 mg/m^2 as a single dose every 3 weeks; 20 mg/m^2 weekly; or 30 mg/m^2/day for 3 days and repeated every 4 weeks.

Route

I.V.

Uses

Treatment of acute lymphoblastic and myeloblastic leukemias, lymphomas, sarcomas, neuroblastomas, and Wilm's tumor.

Interactions

Doxorubicin is incompatible if mixed with heparin or 5-fluorouracil (drug precipitates).

Adverse reactions
Nausea, vomiting, stomatitis, bone marrow depression, fever, local phlebitis, alopecia, and high-dose toxicity (including cardiac abnormalities, EKG changes, and heart failure).

Special considerations
• Use only distilled water as a diluent.
• Administer through a free-flowing infusion to minimize vascular irritation. (Extravasation may not cause pain as a warning signal.)
• Observe for any changes in heart rate or rhythm and signs of heart failure.
• Total dose must not exceed 550 mg/m².
• Warn child and caregivers that drug causes urine to turn red (for up to 12 days after administration); this discoloration is a normal reaction, not an indication of hematuria.

Hydroxyurea (Hydrea)
Dosage
20 to 30 mg/kg/day on a continual basis.
Route
P.O.
Uses
Treatment of sarcomas, lymphomas, and leukemia.
Interactions
None known.
Adverse reactions
Nausea, vomiting, and anorexia; less commonly: diarrhea, bone marrow depression, mucosal ulceration, alopecia, and dermatitis.
Special considerations
• Give drug cautiously to patients with renal dysfunction.
• Severe erythema may occur if used in combination with radiation therapy.

Lomustine (CeeNU)
Dosage
130 mg/m² as a single dose every 6 weeks. Reduce dose according to bone marrow depression.
Route
P.O.
Uses
Treatment of brain tumors and neuroblastomas.
Interactions
None known.
Adverse reactions
Nausea and vomiting (usually within 2 to 6 hours), bone marrow depression (usually 4 to 6 weeks later).

Special considerations
• Use cautiously if bone marrow depression is already present.
• Drug crosses the blood-brain barrier.
• Administer antiemetics before dose in fasting patients.

Mechlorethamide hydrochloride (Mustargen)

Dosage
0.4 mg/kg as a single dose or divided in 2 to 4 daily doses (0.2 mg/kg or 0.1 mg/kg respectively). Dosage is repeated when child shows evidence of hematologic recovery (usually no earlier than 3 weeks).

Route
I.V. or intrathecal.

Uses
Treatment of Hodgkin's and other lymphomas, neuroblastomas, and retinoblastomas.

Interactions
None known.

Adverse reactions
Nausea and vomiting (usually within ½ to 8 hours), bone marrow depression (usually 2 to 3 weeks later), alopecia, and local phlebitis.

Special considerations
• Use caution in mixing drug. Wear protective eyeglasses or goggles to avoid getting vapors in the eyes; if solution contacts skin, rinse with copious amount of water.
• Drug is unstable once mixed; use immediately.
• Infuse through a free-flowing infusion; extravasation causes skin necrosis and sloughing.
• Irradiation of the sternum, ribs, or vertebrae after a course of mechlorethamide may lead to hematologic complications.

Mercaptopurine (Purinethol)

Dosage
Initially, 2.5 mg/kg/day for several weeks. Maintenance dosage is 1.5 to 2.5 mg/kg/day.

Route
P.O.

Uses
Treatment of acute leukemias.

Interactions
• Delayed metabolism and increased potency occur when used with allopurinol.
• Mercaptopurine is effective when used in combination with methotrexate to treat children with acute lymphatic leukemia in remission.

• Hepatotoxicity occurs when used in combination with doxorubicin.

Adverse reactions
Nausea, vomiting, diarrhea, abdominal pain, anorexia, stomatitis, bone marrow depression (4 to 6 weeks later), immunosuppression, dermatitis, and (less commonly) hepatic dysfunction.

Special considerations
Abdominal pain usually is relieved with defecation.

Methotrexate (Amethopterin)

Dosage
Initially, 3.3 mg/m^2 in combination with 60 mg/m^2 of prednisone. Maintenance dosage (in combination with other agents) varies according to chemotherapy protocol.

Route
P.O., I.V., I.M., or intrathecal.

Uses
Treatment of leukemia, sarcomas, and brain tumors.

Interactions
Salicylates, sulfonamides, phenytoin, phenylbutazone, tetracycline, chloramphenicol, and para-aminobenzoic acid should not be given with methotrexate because of the competition for serum albumin binding.

Adverse reactions
Nausea, vomiting, diarrhea, mucosal ulcerations (2 to 5 days later), bone marrow depression (10 days later), immunosuppression, dermatitis and skin sensitivity to sun, photosenstivity, and (rarely) alopecia; toxic effects: hepatitis (fibrosis), osteoporosis, nephropathy, pneumonitis (fibrosis), and hemorrhagic enteritis.

Special considerations
• Citrovorum factor (folinic acid or leucovorin) decreases cytotoxic action of methotrexate. (Citrovorum—a reduced form of folic acid—is used as an antidote for overdose and to enhance normal cell recovery after intense therapy.) Avoid using vitamins during drug administration, unless prescribed by doctor.
• Intrathecal route is associated with increased toxicity, including pain at injection site, meningismus (signs of meningitis without actual inflammation), fever, headache, and potential sequelae (including transient or permanent hemiparesis, convulsions, dementia, and death).
• Meningeal irritation can be minimized by using a preservative-free diluent, allowing the drug to warm to room temperature before administration, and filtering the drug through a Millipore filter before administration. Use of an Ommaya reservoir also decreases adverse reactions.

Procarbazine hydrochloride (Matulane)

Dosage

Dosage is highly individualized in children. General guidelines include the following: 50 mg/day for 1 week followed by 100 mg/m²/day until maximum response is achieved or leukopenia or thrombocytopenia occurs. Drug is then discontinued until hematologic recovery occurs, then resumed at 50 mg/day and maintained with hematologic monitoring.

Route

P.O.

Uses

Treatment of Hodgkin's and other lymphomas, neuroblastomas, and embryonal carcinomas.

Interactions

• MAO inhibition sometimes occurs; sympathomimetics and such foods as aged cheese, yogurt, alcohol, and bananas should be avoided.

• CNS depressants (such as phenothiazines and barbiturates) enhance CNS symptoms.

Adverse reactions

Severe nausea and vomiting, bone marrow depression (3 to 4 weeks later), lethargy, dermatitis, myalgia, and arthralgia; less commonly: stomatitis, neuropathy, alopecia, and diarrhea.

Special considerations

• Hospitalization usually is required for the initial course if renal or hepatic impairment exist.

• Report any CNS symptoms.

• Observe for hemorrhagic tendencies.

Thioguanine (Thioguan)

Dosage

Used most often in multiple drug protocols. If used alone, dosage is approximately 2 mg/kg/day for 4 weeks; may be increased with caution to 3 mg/kg/day.

Route

P.O.

Uses

Treatment of acute myeloblastic leukemia.

Interactions

• Increased liver toxicity occurs if administered with other potentially hepatotoxic drugs.

• Cross-resistance occurs when used with mercaptopurine.

Adverse reactions

Nausea, vomiting, bone marrow depression, stomatitis, and (rarely) dermatitis, photosensitivity, and liver dysfunction.

Special considerations
• Adverse reactions to drug are uncommon.
• Overdosage may manifest with nausea, vomiting, malaise, hypertension, and diaphoresis. Delayed manifestations of overdosage include myelosuppression and azotemia.

Vinblastine sulfate (Velban)

Dosage
Dosage schedule is as follows:
• First dose: 2.5 mg/m²/week as a single dose.
• Second dose: 3.75 mg/m²/week as a single dose.
• Third dose: 5 mg/m²/week as a single dose.
• Fourth dose: 6.25 mg/m²/week as a single dose.
• Fifth dose: 7.5 mg/m²/week as a single dose.
(*Note:* Maximum dose is 12.5 mg/m². Next higher dose should never be given until white blood cell count has returned to at least 4,000/mm³.)

Route
I.V.

Uses
Treatment of Hodgkin's and other lymphomas.

Interactions
• Potentially neurotoxic drugs must not be given with vinblastine because of neurologic adverse reactions.
• Bronchospasm and acute dyspnea occur if given with mitomycin.

Adverse reactions
Nausea, vomiting, bone marrow depression (especially neutropenia), alopecia, and neurotoxicity (same as for vincristine, but less severe).

Special considerations
• Extravasation causes cellulitis; administer drug through a free-flowing infusion.
• Patients with underlying problems may be prone to neurotoxicity. Report any signs of neurotoxicity; cessation of drug may be required.
• Institute safety precautions (such as use of side rails and a wheelchair and assistance when walking) if patient has impaired ambulation.
• Monitor stool patterns closely.
• Because drug is excreted primarily into the biliary system, administer cautiously to patients with biliary disease.
• Avoid injecting drug into an extremity with poor or potentially impaired circulation; this enhances the risk of thrombosis.
• Fatal if given intrathecally.

Vincristine sulfate (Oncovin)

Dosage
2 mg/m² at weekly intervals.

Route
I.V.

Uses
Treatment of leukemia, Hodgkin's and other lymphomas, Wilms' tumor, neuroblastomas, sarcomas, and brain tumors.

Interactions
See "Vinblastine."

Adverse reactions
Bone marrow depression (especially anemia), alopecia, and neurotoxicity (including paresthesia, ataxia, weakness, footdrop, hyporeflexia, constipation, hoarseness, mental depression, and abdominal, chest, and jaw pain).

Special considerations
See "Vinblastine."

☐ Miscellaneous medications

Acetylcysteine (Mucomyst)

Dosage
1 to 10 ml (20% solution) or 2 to 20 ml (10% solution) every 2 to 6 hours.

Route
Nebulization by mask, mouthpiece, tracheostomy, or Croupette.

Uses
Used as a mucolytic (to liquefy mucus) and as an antidote for acetaminophen overdose.

Interactions
None known.

Adverse reactions
Nausea, vomiting, rash, and bronchoconstriction.

Special considerations
• Maintain fluid intake.
• Be prepared to suction after treatment, especially if cough is inadequate.
• Provide mouth care and wash the child's face after treatment. (Medication feels sticky and has a disagreeable odor.)
• Observe for bronchospasm; bronchodilator may be required.

Alprostadil (Prostin VR Pediatric)

Dosage
Initially, 0.1 mcg/kg/minute I.V.; increase or decrease dosage (maximum of 0.4 mcg/kg/minute), as necessary, to obtain therapeutic response.

Route
I.V. in a large vein.

Uses
Used to relax smooth muscle of ductus arteriosus; maintains patent ductus arteriosus until corrective surgery can be performed (when survival of infant is dependent on a patent ductus). (See "Congenital heart defects" under the "Cardiovascular and respiratory systems" heading in Section 2.)

Interactions
None known.

Adverse reactions
Apnea, fever, seizures, bradycardia, flushing, and hypertension.

Special considerations
• Monitor arterial pressure and ABG levels during treatment.
• Make sure necessary equipment and personnel for ventilatory assistance is on hand in case apnea occurs.

Furosemide (Lasix)

Dosage
1 to 6 mg/kg/day.

Route
P.O., I.M., or I.V.

Uses
Used to manage CHF, hypertension, and edema.

Interactions
• Increased risk of ototoxicity occurs when given with aminoglycosides.
• Furosemide produces enhanced hypokalemia if given with glucocorticoids and certain antibiotics.

Adverse reactions
Dehydration, hyponatremia, hypokalemia, metabolic alkalosis, and other electrolyte imbalances.

Special considerations
• Monitor intake and output, vital signs, and weight.
• Assess skin turgor.
• If giving orally, administer drug with food or milk.
• Make sure child avoids sudden postural changes.
• Provide a high-potassium diet or potassium supplements, as required.
• Emphasize to the child and caregivers the importance of reporting signs and symptoms of hypokalemia (weakness, cramps, dizziness, or nausea) to the doctor.

Hydralazine hydrochloride (Apresoline)

Dosage
0.75 mg/kg/day to 7.5 mg/kg/day P.O. in four doses. Alternatively, 1.7 to 3.5 mg/kg/day I.M. or I.V. in four to six doses.

Route
P.O., I.M., or I.V.

Uses
Treatment of hypertension and CHF.

Interactions
Hydralazine produces additional hypotensive effect if given with MAO inhibitors or nitrates.

Adverse reactions
Headache, tachycardia, nausea, vomiting, edema, diarrhea, and lupus erythematosus–like symptoms.

Special considerations
• Be sure to give medication consistently on time.
• Monitor vital signs and weight, and assess the skin.
• Make sure the child avoids sudden postural changes.

Indomethacin (Indocin)

Dosage
Dosage is given in three doses at 12- to 24-hour intervals:
• Infants under age 2 days: 0.2 mg/kg followed by two doses of 0.1 mg/kg.
• Infants age 2 to 7 days: Three doses of 0.2 mg/kg.
• Infants over age 7 days: 0.2 mg/kg followed by two doses of 0.25 mg/kg.

Route
I.V.

Uses
Alternative to surgery to manage patent ductus arteriosus by inhibition of prostaglandin synthesis.

Interactions
Indomethacin increases digoxin levels. Hyperkalemia may occur if given with potassium-sparing diuretics.

Adverse reactions
Bleeding problems (especially GI and pulmonary); may mask infections.

Special considerations
• Monitor infants on digitalis for signs of toxicity.
• Observe stools for blood.
• Use small-gauge needles for all injections.
• Monitor intake and output carefully.
• Protect infants receiving this drug from infection.

Lactulose (Cephulac, Chronulac)

Dosage
20 to 30 g P.O. three or four times a day; if given rectally, must be diluted and given as a retention enema.

Route
P.O. or rectal.

Uses
Used in renal failure to increase water content of the stool and inhibit diffusion of ammonia from the bowel to the bloodstream.

Interactions
Diminished effectiveness occurs when used concomitantly with neomycin.

Adverse reactions
Cramps, flatulence, abdominal distention, and diarrhea.

Special considerations
• Observe for improvement in mental status (should be evident within 24 to 28 hours if given P.O. and within 2 hours if given rectally), which demonstrates effectiveness of drug.
• Drug may be given with water, juice, or milk.

Mannitol (Osmitrol)

Dosage
1.5 to 2 g/kg as a 15% to 25% solution.

Route
I.V.

Uses
Reduction of intracranial pressure and treatment of renal failure.

Interactions
Mannitol decreases the effectiveness of lithium by rapid excretion.

Adverse reactions
Serious fluid and electrolyte imbalances and phlebitis at the insertion site.

Special considerations
• Assess intake and output, vital signs, and central venous pressure hourly during administration.
• Monitor for signs of fluid overload or dehydration.
• Assess neurologic status and monitor intracranial pressure readings.
• Avoid infiltration, which may result in tissue necrosis.
• An indwelling urinary catheter should be in place during therapy to monitor output accurately.

Pancreatic enzymes

Dosage
Up to 8 tablets or capsules with each meal, adjusted to the degree of steatorrhea; also, 1 tablet or capsule usually is given with each snack.
Commonly used pancreatic enzymes include the following:

• Cotazyme: Cherry-flavored or regular capsules containing a powder.
• Cotazyme-S: Capsules containing enteric-coated spheres. Coating protects enzyme against inactivation by gastric acidity; enzymes are released in the duodenum.
• Ku-Zyme HP: Capsules containing powder. May result in decreased serum iron response to oral iron supplements.
• Pancrease: Capsules containing coated microspheres. Coating resists gastric inactivation.
• Pancreatin: Tablets.
• Viokase: Powder or tablet form. Dosage in powder form is ¼ teaspoon with meals.

Route
P.O.

Uses
Treatment of pancreatic enzyme deficiency in cystic fibrosis.

Interactions
None except for interaction of iron supplements and Ku-zyme HP (see "Dosage" above).

Adverse reactions
High doses may result in hyperuricemia or hyperuricosuria. Overdose produces nausea and diarrhea. May cause allergic reaction in children with pork allergy.

Special considerations
• Spheres or microspheres should not be crushed or chewed.
• If the child cannot swallow, open capsules containing spheres or microspheres and sprinkle on cold food that does not require chewing, such as applesauce or Jell-o. *Note:* Instruct child to eat food quickly or enzyme will begin to digest food.
• Do not give with hot food (inactivates enzyme) or alkaline food (dissolves protective enteric coating).
• Powders may irritate mucous membranes if inhaled or held in mouth. Inhaled powders may produce asthma attack.

Pancuronium bromide (Pavulon)

Dosage
Highly individualized (test dose is 0.02 mg/kg).

Route
I.V.

Uses
Treatment of refractory status epilepticus and Reye's syndrome.

Interactions
• Inhaled anesthetics potentiate effects.
• Neomycin and magnesium sulfate produce increased action.

Adverse reactions
Respiratory arrest.

Special considerations
• When administering drug, make sure equipment for intubation, artificial respiration, and oxygen therapy is on hand. Also keep anticholinesterase (antidote) available at the patient's bedside.
• Because the child will be totally incapacitated during therapy, he'll require constant nursing intervention to prevent skin breakdown as well as pneumonia and other infection.

Phenazopyridine hydrochloride (Pydirium)

Dosage
12 mg/kg/day in three doses; may be given in combination with an antibacterial, such as sulfisoxazole. Usually given on a short-term basis (approximately 2 days).

Route
P.O.

Uses
Relief of discomfort associated with urinary tract infections; acts as a urinary tract analgesic and an antiseptic.

Interactions
None known.

Adverse reactions
Urine discoloration (orange to red), headache, rash, GI disturbances, and methemoglobinemia.

Special considerations
• Give with meals to reduce GI symptoms.
• Warn child and caregivers about possible staining and urine discoloration. Advise that they protect bedding, clothing, and upholstery from stains.
• Discolored urine will stain fabrics permanently.

Appendices

APPENDIX A: COMMON PEDIATRIC-RELATED ABBREVIATIONS

The following list of abbreviations are commonly used on the medical records of pediatric patient.

ADD	Attention deficit disorder
AGN	Acute glomerulonephritis
AIDS	Acquired immunodeficiency syndrome
ALL	Acute lymphocytic leukemia
AML	Acute myelocytic or myeloblastic leukemia
ARF	Acute rheumatic fever
ASD	Atrial septal defect
ASO	Antistreptolysin O
AV	Atrioventricular
BAER	Brainstem auditory evoked response
BOM	Bilateral otitis media
BPD	Bronchopulmonary dysplasia
BRAT	Bananas, rice, applesauce, and toast
BSA	Body surface area
CC	Chest circumference or chief complaint
CF	Cystic fibrosis
CHD	Congenital heart disease
CHF	Congestive heart failure
CL	Cleft lip
CLP	Cleft lip and palate
CMS	Children's medical services
CMV	Cytomegalovirus
CP	Cleft palate or cerebral palsy
CPT	Chest physiotherapy
DDST	Denver Developmental Screening Test
DES	Diethylstilbestrol
DFA	Diet for age
DIC	Disseminated intravascular coagulation
DOE	Dyspnea on exertion
DTP	Diphtheria, tetanus, and pertussis
EBV	Epstein-Barr virus
EES	Erythromycin ethylsuccinate
ESR	Erythrocyte sedimentation rate
ESRD	End-stage renal disease
FAS	Fetal alcohol syndrome
FB	Foreign body
FTT	Failure to thrive
FUO	Fever of unknown origin
G&D	Growth and development
GER	Gastroesophageal reflux
G_6PD	Glucose-6-phosphate dehydrogenase
GFR	Glomerular filtration rate
HBO	Hyperbaric oxygen
HC	Head circumference
HIB	*Hemophilus influenzae,* type B
HIV	Human immunodeficiency virus
HRS	Health and rehabilitative services
IAC	Idiopathic anemia of childhood
IDDM	Insulin-dependent diabetes mellitus
IPV	Inactivated poliovirus vaccine (Salk)
ISADH	Inappropriate secretion of anti-diuretic hormone
JRA	Juvenile rheumatoid arthritis
LBW	Low birth weight
LGA	Large for gestational age
LLL	La Leche league
LTB	Laryngotracheobronchitis
MI	Mitral insufficiency
MMR	Measles, mumps, and rubella
MR	Mental retardation
MS	Mitral stenosis
NEC	Necrotizing enterocolitis
NHL	Non-Hodgkin's lymphoma
NICU	Neonatal intensive care unit
MCT	Medium chain triglycerides
OM	Otitis media
O&P	Ova and parasites
OPV	Oral polio vaccine
PD	Postural drainage
PDA	Patent ductus arteriosus
PFC	Persistent fetal circulation
PI	Pulmonary insufficiency
PICU	Pediatric intensive care unit
PKU	Phenylketonuria
PMI	Point of maximum impulse
PS	Pulmonic stenosis
PVD	Percussion, vibration, and drainage
RAP	Recurrent abdominal pain
RDS	Respiratory distress syndrome
RF	Rheumatic fever
RLF	Retrolental fibroplasia
RSV	Respiratory syncytial virus
SDF	Safe dose factor
SGA	Small for gestational age
SIDS	Sudden infant death syndrome
SISADH	Syndrome of inappropriate secretion of anti-diuretic hormone
SOM	Serous otitis media
STD	Sexually transmitted disease
T&A	Tonsillectomy and adenoidectomy
TEF	Tracheoesophageal fistula
TEV	Talipes equinovarus
TIBC	Total iron-binding capacity
TLC	Tender loving care
TOPV	Trivalent oral polio vaccine (Sabin)
TPN	Total parenteral nutrition
VSD	Ventricular septal defect

APPENDIX B: TERMINOLOGY

Achondroplasia Dwarfism resulting from inadequate enchondral bone formation. May be nutritional or congenital in etiology.

Aniridia Absence of the iris

Apgar score A numerical rating of the condition of a newborn infant based on points assigned for heart rate, respiratory status, color, muscle tone, and reflex irritability. Best possible score is 10.

Arnold-Chiari malformation A congenital displacement of the brain stem and cerebellum through the foramen magnum. May be associated with spina bifida.

Beau's lines Furrows occurring transversely on fingernails following a wasting disease.

Blount's disease Lateral bowing of the leg from aseptic necrosis of the medial tibial condyle.

Bruxism Unconscious grinding of the teeth, especially during periods of sleep or stress.

Cholesteatoma A mass comprised of cholesterol and epithelial cells commonly found in the middle ear. May occur as a complication of chronic otitis media or as a congenital problem.

Cri-du-chat Literally, "cry of cat". A high-pitched meowing cry associated with a congenital disorder that includes numerous anomalies.

Crohn's disease Chronic inflammatory disease of the bowel of unknown etiology.

Curling's ulcer A duodenal ulcer occurring in association with severe burns of the skin.

Encopresis Fecal incontinence.

Enuresis Incontinence of urine.

Extrusion reflex Outward protrusion of the infant's tongue when it is touched. Normally disappears at age 3 to 4 months.

Floppy baby A term generally used to describe an infant with poor muscle tone. Floppy infant syndromes—inherited neuromuscular disorders, including Werdnig-Hoffman paralysis and Wohlfart-Kugelberg-Welander disease.

Gilles de la Tourette syndrome A condition characterized by involuntary movements and speech.

Hemosiderosis A condition characterized by excessive iron stores in various organs of the body, often associated with chronic hemolytic disorders.

Henoch-Schönlein purpura An analphylactic response characterized by vasculitis, purpuric skin lesions, hematuria, and GI bleeding.

Heptavax-B Vaccine against hepatitis B.

Macewan's sign "Cracked pot" sound obtained upon percussion of the skull of a hydrocephalic child.

Marasmus A condition of severe wasting occurring as a result of physical and/or emotional deprivation and occasionally caused by a metabolic defect.

Menarche Onset of menstruation.

Olive sign Mass of hypertrophic pyloric sphincter palpable through the abdominal wall.

Pica Cravings for and ingestion of unusual and unnatural substances.

Setting sun sign "Sunset eyes." Sclera above the iris is visible. Seen in conditions such as hydrocephalus.

Sprue Celiac disease. A chronic malabsorptive disease characterized by steatorrhea, abdominal distention, and malnutrition.

Stevens-Johnson syndrome   A form of erythema multiforme, with fever and erosive lesions of ecto-dermal tissues (e.g., skin, mucous membranes, and nervous system). May be a reaction to sulfonamide therapy.

Talipes equinovarus   An inversion deformity of the foot in which the forefoot is adducted so there is plantar flexion. Also called clubfoot.

Tanner staging   A system for describing the developmental stages of secondary sex characteristics.

Tay-Sachs disease   An inherited disorder occurring most commonly in children of Eastern European Jewish families. It is marked by mental retardation, blind-ness, paralysis, and early death. There is no known treatment.

Thelarche   Beginning of breast development.

Turner's syndrome   A congenital syndrome of females characterized by the absence of an X chromosone and varying degrees of learning disorders. Therapy is largely hormonal.

Tympanometry   A measurement of the compliance of the ear drum using special equipment. Useful for the detection of middle ear effusion and scar-ring or rupture of the tympanic membrane, especially when visualiza-tion is not possible.

Washington Guide   A tool to guide in the promotion of development in the child from age 1 to 52 months. Expected tasks are listed with suggested activities for developmental achievement.

APPENDIX C: PHYSICAL GROWTH CHARTS

To use the growth charts* on the following pages, correlate the child's age with the appropriate growth measurement (head circumference, length/height, or weight). Consider the child's growth normal if the plotted measurement falls between the 5th and 95th percentiles; consider the child's growth abnormal if it falls below the 5th or above the 95th percentile.

Boys: birth to 36 months

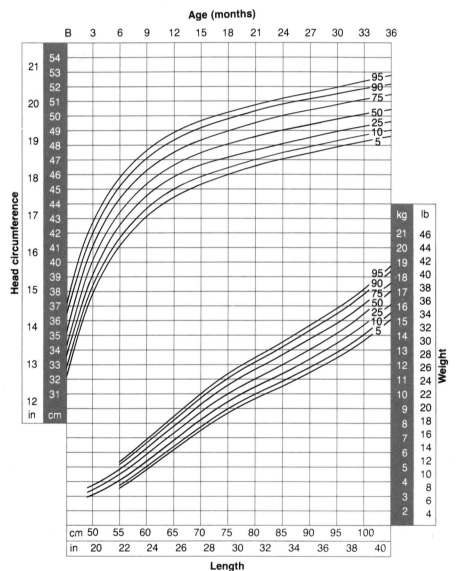

*Adapted from National Center for Health Statistics. *NCHS Growth Charts,* Rockville, Md., 1976.

PHYSICAL GROWTH CHARTS *(continued)*

Girls: birth to 36 months

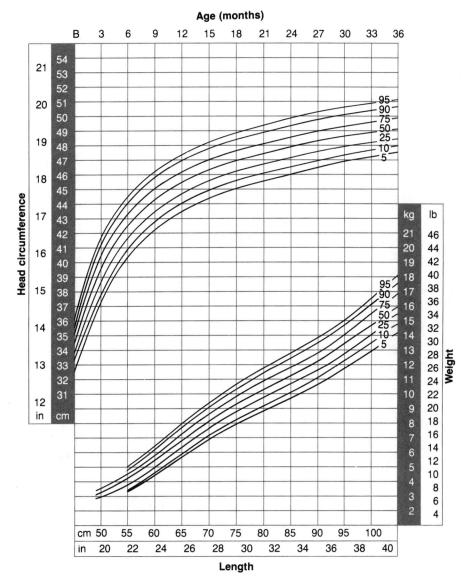

(continued)

PHYSICAL GROWTH CHARTS *(continued)*

Boys: 2 to 18 years

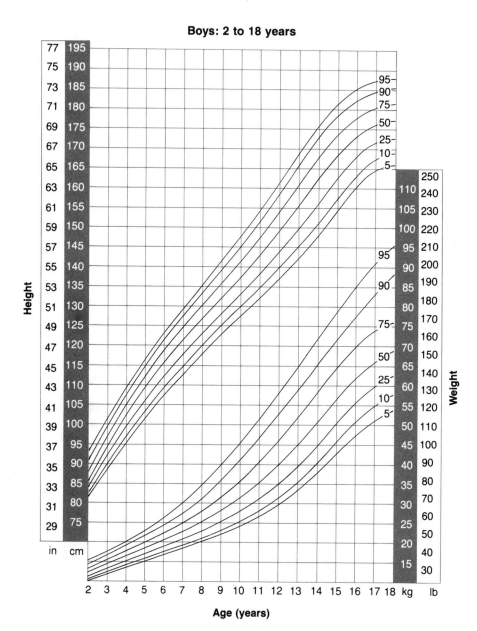

Age (years)

PHYSICAL GROWTH CHARTS *(continued)*

Girls: 2 to 18 years

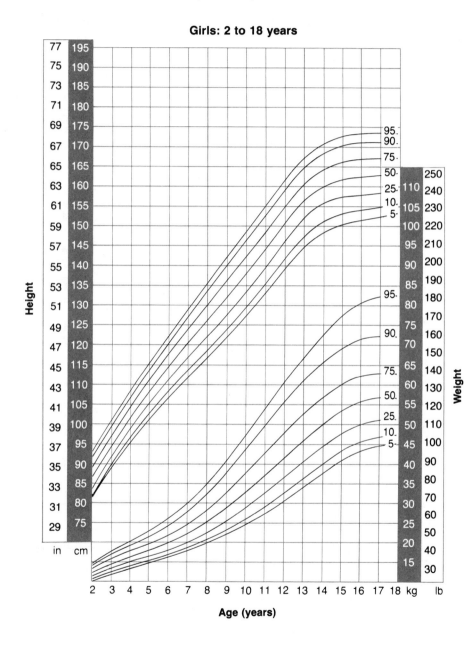

Height

Weight

Age (years)

APPENDIX D: FLUID AND ELECTROLYTE IMBALANCE

Below is a listing of some of the most common types of primary disturbances in fluids and electrolytes along with common causes, signs and symptoms, and laboratory findings.

Type of disturbance	Causes	Signs and symptoms	Laboratory findings
FLUID IMBALANCES			
Interstitial-to-plasma fluid shift	• Recovery from plasma-to-interstitial shift (such as occurs with recovery from burns) • Volume replacement after hypovolemia (such as after hemorrhage or the administration of excessive amounts of blood, plasma, blood expanders, or hypertonic solutions)	Signs and symptoms of hypervolemia, including bounding pulse, peripheral vein engorgement, moist crackles, weakness, pallor, and hyperpnea	Decreased red blood cell (RBC) count, packed cell volume, and hemodilution
Plasma-to-interstitial fluid shift	• Portal hypertension (such as in chronic liver disease) • Decreased oncotic pressure with increased capillary permeability (such as from malnutrition, starvation edema, burns, crushing injuries, or nephrotic syndrome) • Vasodilation (such as from shock) • Decreased venous return	Ascites, peripheral edema, and signs of hypovolemia (including pallor, tachycardia, low blood pressure, weak pulse, cold extremities, and disorientation)	Elevated hematocrit level, RBC count, and packed cell volume
Water depletion	• Inadequate water intake (from total cessation of intake or prolonged diminished intake) • Failure to absorb or reabsorb water (such as from diarrhea or an intestinal disorder) • Water loss from the GI tract (such as from vomiting, diarrhea, fistula, or nasogastric suction) • Excessive renal excretion (such as in inappropriate secretion of antidiuretic hormone, diabetes mellitus, or renal disease) • Iatrogenic causes (such as from overuse of diuretics or improper postoperative fluid replacement) • Impaired skin integrity (such as from burns, wounds, or hemorrhage)	Thirst, variable temperature, dry skin and mucous membranes, poor skin turgor, weight loss, fatigue, oliguria, depressed fontanelles, irritability, lethargy, and sunken eyeballs; severe symptoms: signs of shock, soft eyeballs, rapid pulse and respiratory rates, and low blood pressure	High urine specific gravity (except in inappropriate secretion of antidiuretic hormone), increased blood urea nitrogen level, variable serum sodium concentration, normal or increased potassium level, and increased hematocrit level
Water excess	• Water intake in excess of output (such as from excessive oral intake, overloading with hypotonic solution, and administration of plain water enemas) • Failure to excrete water while maintaining normal intake (such as in kidney disease, congestive heart failure, or malnutrition)	Edema, moist crackles, loose aerolar tissues of the eyelids and scotum, elevated venous pressure, bradycardia, weight gain, lethargy, increased spinal fluid pressure, convulsions, and coma	Low urine specific gravity, dilution of electrolytes, decreased hematocrit level, variable urine volume, and hemodilution

FLUID AND ELECTROLYTE IMBALANCE *(continued)*

Type of disturbance	Causes	Signs and symptom	Laboratory findings
ELECTROLYTE IMBALANCES			
Hypercalcemia (calcium excess)	• Calcium converted from nonionized to ionized (as in acidosis, prolonged immobilization, or conditions associated with increased bone catabolism) • Inadequate elimination (as in kidney disease) • Increased absorption of calcium from the GI tract (such as with hypervitaminosis D) • Increased resorption of calcium by the kidneys (as in hyperparathyroidism)	Constipation, anorexia, mouth dryness, muscle hypotonicity, and kidney stones resulting from increased urine calcium concentrations	Increased calcium concentration in the urine
Hypocalcemia (calcium depletion)	• Inadequate intake (as in low-calcium diet) • Malabsorption from GI tract (as in vitamin D deficiency or rapid transit through the GI tract) • Excessive calcium losses (such as in advanced renal insufficiency or hypoparathyroidism) • Decreased bone resorption (as in alkalosis) • Unavailability for use as ionized calcium (such as calcium trapped in diseased tissues, tetany of the newborn from cow's milk formula, or exchange transfusion with titrated blood)	Neuromuscular irritability; tingling of the nose, ears, fingertips, and toes; tetany; laryngospasm; generalized convulsions; possible changes in clotting; positive Chvostek's sign; and cardiac arrest	Calcium level less than 4.5 mEq/liter
Hyperchloremia (chloride excess)	• Excessive ingestion (such as in treatments using ammonium chloride) • Decreased output (such as in renal disease)	Tachypnea, weakness, and symptoms associated with acidosis	Low carbon dioxide combining power
Hypochloremia (chloride depletion)	• Inadequate intake (such as in starvation or inadequate replacement of losses) • Excessive excretion (such as with vomiting, pyloric stenosis, or nasogastric suction)	Symptoms associated with alkalosis (including lethargy and muscle hypertonicity), depressed respirations, and metabolic alkalosis	Chloride level less than 100 mEq/liter, high carbon dioxide combining power

(continued)

FLUID AND ELECTROLYTE IMBALANCE *(continued)*

Type of disturbance	Causes	Signs and symptom	Laboratory findings
ELECTROLYTE IMBALANCES (continued)			
Hyperkalemia (potassium excess)	• Inadequate excretion (such as in renal disease, renal shutdown, adrenal insufficiency, or metabolic acidosis) • Increased intake (such as from too-rapid administration of potassium chloride I.V.) • Movement from intracellular to extracellular fluid (such as in severe dehydration, crushing injuries, burns, or hemolysis from sudden massive water intake) • Hemoconcentration (such as in dehydration)	Muscle weakness, flaccid paralysis, twitching, hyperreflexia, bradycardia, ventricular fibrillation and cardiac arrest, oliguria, and apnea (respiratory arrest)	High serum potassium concentration, variable urine volume, flat P waves on EKG
Hypokalemia (potassium depletion)	• Inadequate potassium intake (such as in starvation or with inadequate amounts of potassium added to I.V. solutions) • Loss from GI tract (such as from vomiting, diarrhea, fistulas, or nasogastric suction) • Excessive renal excretion (such as with diuresis, administration of diuretics, administration of corticosteroids, the diuretic phase of nephrotic syndrome, the healing stage of burns, potassium-losing nephritis, or hyperglycemic diuresis) • Movement from extracellular to intracellular fluid (such as with alkalosis or the I.V. administration of insulin in ketosis)	Muscle weakness, stiffness, paralysis, or hyporeflexia; hypotension, cardiac dysrhythmias, gallop rhythms, tachycardia or bradycardia, ileus, apathy, drowsiness, irritability, and fatigue	Potassium levels less than 4.1 mEq/liter, decreased serum potassium concentration, and abnormal EKG findings (flat T waves and prolonged ST segments)
Hypernatremia (sodium excess)	• Increased sodium intake without increased output (such as with high-sodium nasogastric or I.V. intake) • Decreased output (as in renal disease)	Intense thirst, dry sticky mucous membranes, flushed skin, possible increased temperature, hoarseness, oliguria, nausea, vomiting, firm tissue turgor, irritability, and possible progression to disorientation and convulsions	Increased or normal serum sodium concentration, high plasma volume, and alkalosis

FLUID AND ELECTROLYTE IMBALANCE *(continued)*

Type of disturbance	Causes	Signs and symptom	Laboratory findings
ELECTROLYTE IMBALANCES (continued)			
Hyponatremia (sodium depletion)	• Inadequate sodium intake (such as from a prolonged low-sodium diet) • Loss through perspiration (such as in fever, excessive sweating, or cystic fibrosis) • Loss through nonintact skin (such as in burns and wounds) • Loss through the GI tract (such as from vomiting, diarrhea, nasogastric suction, or fistulas) • Excessive renal excretion (such as in adrenal insufficiency) • Associated with water deficit or excess (such as in renal disease or diabetic acidosis)	When associated with water loss: same symptoms as with water loss (including dehydration, weakness, dizziness, nausea, abdominal cramps, and apprehension); with mild depletion: apathy, weakness, nausea, and weak pulse; with moderate depletion: decreased blood pressure	Variable sodium concentration (may be high, low, or normal), and variable urine specific gravity (depending on water deficit or excess). Normal serum sodium level is 135 to 145 mEq/liter.

APPENDIX E: CLINICAL SIGNS OF DEHYDRATION

The following groupings show clinical signs and symptoms for three types of dehydration.

Isotonic (sodium and water depletion)	Hypotonic (sodium depletion in excess of water)	Hypertonic (water depletion in excess of sodium)
• Cold, dry, grayish skin with poor turgor	• Cold, clammy, grayish skin with extremely poor turgor	• Cold or hot, thickened, grayish skin with fair turgor
• Dry mucous membranes	• Slightly moist mucous membranes	• Parched mucous membranes
• No tears or salivation	• No tears or salivation	• No tears or salivation
• Sunken, soft eyeballs	• Sunken, soft eyeballs	• Sunken eyeballs
• Sunken fontanelles	• Sunken fontanelles	• Sunken fontanelles
• Subnormal or elevated temperature	• Abnormal temperature	• Subnormal or elevated temperature
• Rapid pulse rate	• Extremely rapid pulse rate	• Moderately rapid pulse rate
• Rapid respiratory rate	• Rapid respiratory rate	• Rapid respiratory rate
• Irritable to lethargic behavior	• Lethargic to comatose behavior; possible convulsions	• Markedly lethargic behavior with extreme hyperirritability on stimulation

APPENDIX F: NANDA TAXONOMY OF NURSING DIAGNOSES

A taxonomy for discussing nursing diagnoses has evolved over several years. The following list contains the approved diagnostic labels of the North American Nursing Diagnosis Association (NANDA), as of summer 1988.

Activity intolerance
Activity intolerance: Potential
Adjustment, impaired
Airway clearance, ineffective
Anxiety
Aspiration, potential for
Body temperature, altered: Potential
Bowel elimination, altered: Colonic constipation
Bowel elimination, altered: Constipation
Bowel elimination, altered: Diarrhea
Bowel elimination, altered: Incontinence
Bowel elimination, altered: Perceived constipation
Breast-feeding, ineffective
Breathing pattern, ineffective
Cardiac output, altered: Decreased
Comfort, altered: Chronic pain
Comfort, altered: Pain
Communication, impaired: Verbal
Coping, family: Potential for growth
Coping, ineffective: Defensive
Coping, ineffective: Denial
Coping, ineffective family: Compromised
Coping, ineffective individual
Decisional conflict (specify)
Disuse syndrome, potential for
Diversional activity, deficit
Dysreflexia
Family processes, altered
Fatigue
Fear
Fluid volume deficit: Actual (1)
Fluid volume deficit: Actual (2)
Fluid volume deficit: Potential
Fluid volume excess
Gas exchange, impaired
Grieving, anticipatory
Grieving, dysfunctional
Growth and development, altered
Health maintenance, altered
Health-seeking behaviors (specify)
Home maintenance management, impaired
Hopelessness
Hyperthermia
Hypothermia
Incontinence, functional
Incontinence, reflex
Incontinence, stress
Incontinence, total

APPENDIX F: NANDA TAXONOMY OF NURSING DIAGNOSES
(continued)

Incontinence, urge
Infection, potential for
Injury, potential for
Injury, potential for: Poisoning
Injury, potential for: Suffocating
Injury, potential for: Trauma
Knowledge deficit (specify)
Mobility, impaired physical
Noncompliance (specify)
Nutrition, altered: Less than body requirements
Nutrition, altered: More than body requirements
Nutrition, altered: Potential for more than body requirements
Parental role, conflict
Parenting, altered: Actual
Parenting, altered: Potential
Post-trauma response
Powerlessness
Rape-trauma syndrome
Rape-trauma syndrome: Compound reaction
Rape-trauma syndrome: Silent reaction
Role performance, altered
Self-care deficit: Bathing and hygiene
Self-care deficit: Dressing and grooming
Self-care deficit: Feeding
Self-care deficit: Toileting
Self-concept, disturbance in: Body image
Self-concept, disturbance in: Personal identity
Self-esteem, chronic low
Self-esteem, disturbance in
Self-esteem, situational low
Sensory-perceptual alteration: Visual, auditory, kinesthetic, gustatory, tactile, olfactory
Sexual dysfunction
Sexuality, altered patterns
Skin integrity, impaired: Actual
Skin integrity, impaired: Potential
Sleep pattern disturbance
Social interaction, impaired
Social isolation
Spiritual distress (distress of the human spirit)
Swallowing, impaired
Thermoregulation, ineffective
Thought processes, altered
Tissue integrity, impaired
Tissue integrity, impaired: Oral mucous membrane
Tissue perfusion, altered: Renal, cerebral, cardiopulmonary, gastrointestinal, peripheral
Unilateral neglect
Urinary elimination, altered patterns
Urinary retention
Violence, potential for: Self-directed or directed at others

Selected References

Books

DeAngelis, C. *Pediatric Primary Care*. Boston: Little, Brown & Co., 1984.

Evans, M.L., and Hansen, B.D. *Guide to Pediatric Nursing: A Clinical Reference*. East Norwalk, Conn.: Appleton & Lange, 1980.

Ingalls, A., and Salverno, M. *Maternal and Child Health Nursing*. St. Louis: C.V. Mosby Co., 1983.

Lesner, P. *Pediatric Nursing*. New York: Delmar Publishers, 1983.

Malasanos, L., et al. *Health Assessment*. St. Louis: C.V. Mosby Co., 1986.

Neurologic Disorders. Nurse's Clinical Library. Springhouse, Pa.: Springhouse Corp., 1984.

Nursing Pediatric Patients. Nursing Photobook Series. Springhouse, Pa.: Springhouse Corp., 1983.

Pediatric Care. Clinical Pocket Manual Series. Springhouse, Pa.: Springhouse Corp., 1987.

Steele, S. *Child Health and the Family: Nursing Concepts and Management*. New York: Masson, 1981.

Ulrich, S., et al. *Nursing Care Planning Guides*. Philadelphia: W.B. Saunders Co., 1986.

Whaley, L., and Wong, D. *Nursing Care of Infants and Children*. St. Louis: C.V. Mosby Co., 1983.

Wong, D., and Whaley, L. *Clinical Handbook of Pediatric Nursing*. St. Louis: C.V. Mosby Co., 1981.

Periodicals

Barnes, C., et al. "The Child with Failure to Thrive," *Pediatric Nursing Forum* 1(1):3-10, 1986.

Colabro, J. "Kawasaki Disease: Inscrutable and Unmistakeable," *Emergency Medicine* 14(2):24-34, 1982.

Gaylord, N., and Carson, S. "Abdominal Pain in Children," *Nurse Practitioner* 8(8):19-24, 1983.

Gretz, K., et al. "Pediatric AIDS: Nursing Care of the Child and Family," *Pediatric Nursing Forum* 3(1), 1988.

Habal, M. "The Team Approach: Comprehensive Care of Patients Born with Cleft Lips and/or Cleft Palates," *Pediatric Basics—Gerber Medical Services* 45, 1986.

Other

Audio-Digest Foundation. *Audio-Digest Pediatrics (1987-1988)*. Glendale, Calif., 1988.

Index

i refers to an illustration; t refers to a table

i refers to an illustration; t refers to a table

i refers to an illustration; t refers to a table

Notes

Notes

Notes